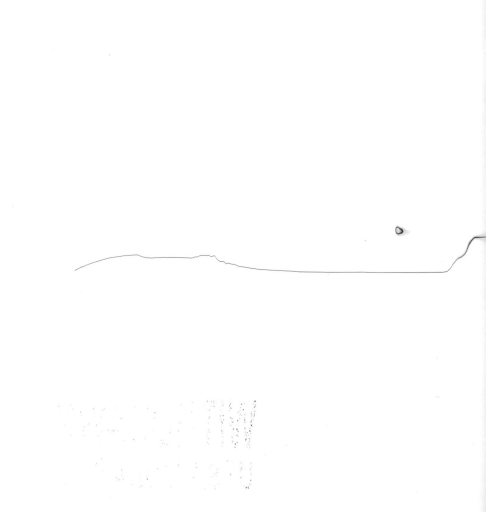

The Yipping Tiger

The Yipping Tiger

and other tales from the neuropsychiatric clinic

Perminder Sachdev, M.D.

The Johns Hopkins University Press
Baltimore

To my parents

Published in Australia by University of New South Wales Press Ltd.

First published in the United States in 2009 by the Johns Hopkins University Press.

9 8 7 6 5 4 3 2 1

The Johns Hopkins University Press
2715 N. Charles Street
Baltimore, Maryland 21218-4363
www.press.jhu.edu

Library of Congress Control Number: 2009929221

ISBN 13: 978-0-8018-9454-1
ISBN 10: 0-8018-9454-9

Design Josephine Pajor-Markus
Printer KHL Printing Co Pte Ltd, Singapore

This book is printed on paper using fibre supplied from plantation or sustainably managed forests.

Contents

Preface

This book is about the marvel called the brain. If evolution is the greatest miracle of nature, the human brain is the pinnacle of its glory. As mankind ventures further into the stars, it is the human brain that enables us to explore the mysteries of the universe. Throughout history, the human brain has been the agent for immense good as well as unspeakable evil. The most astonishing fact is that the human brain has the capacity to peer into itself. Yet, if there is any great unknown that still confronts the brain and challenges its capacity, it is the mystery of the brain itself.

How can one get to know the brain? Neuroscientists provide one answer to this question. They have developed techniques to explore the ultrastructural workings of the brain; its neuroanatomy has been described in exquisite detail, and the complexity of its chemical and electrical transmission continues to challenge our abilities to synthesise and absorb. Its networks are yielding their complexity to persistent scientific enquiry. We now have tools to image the living and working brain with high precision. Since the 1970s we have arguably learnt more about the human brain than in all the preceding centuries. There are more neuroscientists currently alive than have existed in all of history. How far are we then down the road to understanding the brain? The ten case histories presented in this book should make us bow with humility. The human brain will not give away its secrets so easily!

I first became aware of this when I was still a medical student, about three decades ago. I distinctly remember my first visit to the psychiatry ward. The range of mental disturbance took my breath away, and I walked away with the conviction that the brain would finally be understood through the exploration of mental phenomena in their varying shades of deviance. The neurology ward of my hospital did not leave me with the same degree of exhilaration. Neurology three decades ago was generally a staid affair, shackled by its scientific rigour and objectivity. Neurologists had little time for mental phenomena. I decided to go down the psychiatry path. In the late 1970s in New Delhi, this was a distinctly unpopular choice, and many of my teachers and colleagues tried to dissuade me. My first few years in this field were the most awe-inspiring, as the vagaries of the human mind – indeed the human condition – continued to enthral me. After about three years, some regret was beginning to seep in. I had come to the realisation that just as the neurology of my training years was mindless, the psychiatry I had adopted as my profession was largely brainless. The two disciplines had created a gulf between them and, in the interest of protecting their boundaries, had created high fences where none should exist. The mind and the brain had been locked in separate camps. For me to reach the brain, I had to start with the mind. I had to discover a passage between the two camps.

My opportunity came when I moved to the Neuropsychiatric Institute (NPI) in Sydney in 1987. The NPI was the final port of call for all that was weird and wonderful in psychiatry and neurology. Patients came to the NPI to be assessed and analysed, and the interdisciplinary battles that were still being fought between psychiatry and neurology in most medical schools had been quietly abandoned. The brain was always the stage on which the mental theatre was performed. The acts were sometimes mental, at other times neurological, but always neuropsychiatric. It may seem strange that in the twenty-first century we are still talking about the mind and brain as if they are distinct entities. The great advances in cognitive neuroscience of the later twentieth century have challenged the distinction between mental and neural, and the rationale for the division between psychiatric and neurological has been eroded. Yet we remain simplistic – even primitive – in some of our concepts, and continue to treat psychological and organic or mental and physical as being categorically distinct.

The case studies that comprise this book are gems from the rich pickings in the clinic I have run at the NPI for 20 years. They were selected primarily for their ability to inform us about the workings of the brain. The clinical descriptions are interspersed with commentary and dialogue, and peppered with other examples. The final presentation may therefore not simulate what exactly transpired in the clinical encounters. At times some literary concessions have been taken but without compromising scientific accuracy or clinical authenticity. I could be accused of some embellishment, but the stories are based on real patients whose identities have been completely camouflaged to protect their privacy. I justify the literary touch-up for the simple reason that these stories are addressed to a lay audience and not a scientific journal.

If the reader, after having read this book, walks away with

wonderment about the brain, my objective would be fulfilled. If he or she is also amazed and enthralled by the human condition that these cases present, my joy would be boundless. In their brain–mind foibles, I hope to have captured some of their humanity in all its frailty and emotion-laden sanity. We are not human if we are perfect. We may strive to be, but it is my belief – should I even say 'hope' – that we will never attain that goal.

The titles of the chapters may seem enigmatic, but each has a reference to a neuropsychiatric syndrome. They can be decoded as follows:

1	The Yipping Tiger	Golfer's cramps
2	Shaking hands with Dr Strangelove	The alien hand syndrome
3	Swearing like a Spanish sailor	Coprolalia in Tourette's syndrome
4	The Mozart complex	Brain enhancement
5	The mirror always lies	Anorexia nervosa
6	The dead homunculus	Frontal lobe dysfunction
7	Serotonin's seductive song	Major depression
8	A chesty problem	Obsessive-compulsive disorder
9	Lord Nelson's ghost	Phantom limb
10	Freudian slips and semantic slides	Mild cognitive impairment

My journey in this book has seen many companions, but these ten have been constant and deserve my greatest gratitude. There have been numerous other patients and colleagues who have challenged and informed, the majority of whom will remain anonymous. Their generosity towards me knows no bounds. A constant source of inspiration and support through the writing of this book has been my partner for life, Jagdeep, whose sharp clinical mind has often prevented me from drifting too far into academic detail. My *joie de vivre* is my two daughters, Sonal and Nupur, who have such beautiful brains. My particular thanks go to Angela Russell, my editorial assistant and colleague, who spent many days poring over my editorial shortcomings. My gratitude also goes to my colleague Dr Julian Trollor, who has been a companion through the neuropsychiatric journey for 14 years, and to Professor Gordon Parker for his wisdom and guiding generosity through my career. I would like to thank Dr Lubna McDonald for her incisive comments on the first few chapters. The University of New South Wales has provided an excellent platform for my work, and the Prince of Wales Hospital has given me the opportunity to indulge my curiosity. Finally, I salute all my colleagues in the international neuropsychiatric community – they are all brave actors on the stage of the brain–mind theatre.

1

The Yipping Tiger

Was there ever a greater affliction?

An affected golfer

The golf swing is an act of grace and supreme poise. It is also one of the most accurate, smoothly coordinated and ultimately reproducible motor acts. An enthusiastic golfer, driving a tiny ball (42.67 mm, weighing less than 45.93 g) down a sly green toward an elusive hole (10.795 cm), does not perhaps realise that the stroke he or she executes in a fraction of a second is the result of the coordinated action of hundreds of muscles, all orchestrated to the finest degree to the tune of play. There are muscles to maintain the general stance of the body, muscles to fixate the head and the gaze on the ball, muscles to keep some joints immobile, muscles to produce the movement in the right direction at the right speed with the right force, muscles to see that the others do not overshoot the mark, and muscles to follow through. The complexity of a Mozart symphony pales in comparison. Yet the golf stroke is executed so effortlessly, at the same time taking into consideration the unevenness of the green, the moisture left by the overnight rain and the easterly breeze or the southerly storm. What part of the brain conducts this orchestra so masterfully, and how does it do so? If there is indeed a 'golf conductor' in the brain, where is it located and how does it come to be there? Are some individuals born with the seed for such a conductor? What happens to this conductor when a master starts missing the putts that an amateur sinks with smiling ease?

I first came face to face with these questions when I saw Henry P. in my clinic. It was a peculiar consultation, as Henry walked in without a referral note and declared that he knew there was nothing wrong with him medically. But could I help his golf? Not ever having played a round of golf myself, I was nonplussed. I had known golfers for their single-minded devotion to the game, most of whom regarded Haskell's invention of the rubber golf ball as the greatest invention of all time. They had some famous forebears who exemplified this obsession. Mary, Queen of Scots, possibly the first female golfer, was charged with playing golf in the fields beside Seton only a few days after the murder of her husband. Scotland's King James VI was so zealous in protecting the Scottish heritage of the game that he forbade the purchase of balls from Holland. Was Henry P. in the same mould, so much so that his common sense had parted him? He seemed a congenial sort of fellow, so I decided to humour him.

His problem, he said, was that he suffered from the 'yips'. 'I am a scratch player,[1] with one ambition in life – to make my mark as a professional golfer. I started playing when I was 10, and I've won tournaments over the years. I was one of the best junior golfers in the country. I was set to turn pro until it happened about a year ago … I got the yips. The dreams of challenging Tiger Woods quickly deteriorated into nightmares of yipped putts.[2] My family calls me the Yipping Tiger, and that's not much of a roar!'

His was a curious affliction. Henry had no problems on his practice greens, and he spent hours every day practising his strokes. 'There couldn't be anything wrong with my muscles or my coordination, for I have no trouble sinking the most difficult putts when I am practising on my own. But come a tournament and it's a different story. I can still play the rest of my game quite effortlessly, but soon as I come within 6 feet of the hole, I just fall apart. My arms refuse to obey me. Sometimes I freeze in my putting stance, with the putter glued to the ground and refusing to budge. If I do manage to get it going, the smoothness of the stroke is replaced by a jerky finish. I have started, on occasion, with a 3-foot putt on a level green and ended up with a 15-footer. I could kill myself for that … If I don't do something about it, I'm finished.'

Henry first noticed that something could be wrong during a tournament in the United States, which he 'had to win in order to continue my golf'. He missed four easy putts in one round in a manner that surprised everybody. Initially it was put down to 'a bad day'. 'I had been under a lot of financial strain. My fiancée back home wasn't helping matters by insisting that we set a date for marriage. So I thought that things would get better.' But things only got worse. The problem recurred with regularity, and almost every competitive game was affected.

'Putting used to be my strength. Now I began to dread this stroke … even avoid it if I could. Then I'd have one good day, and hoped it had all gone. No, not really. It came back and it began to haunt me. Initially I did not admit it to myself. I suppose it is the same with all good golfers. The word "yips" is dreaded in the clubhouse. No one dare mention it, for it is bad luck. Maybe it is even contagious, for once they suspect that you have the yips, your golfing partners start shunning you. When I realised that I could not beat the problem on my own, I went to a professional. His response was characteristic … it was my technique and my attitude. So began expensive sessions to improve both; sessions I could not afford, yet had to have. His theory was simple … "You become too anxious as you approach the hole"; "It's because you don't trust yourself"; "You worry too much about what others might think if you missed a lousy putt any fool should sink." But I don't think his theory worked, for I did not get better. It also did not feel right. If I was a nervous person, why was I not nervous when executing the other strokes? Why had it happened to me at the age of 26 when I had been playing golf for 16 years? I had not changed as a person; my attitude to the game has always been as competitive as it is now …

'I'd heard about other golfers who had this problem. The great Ben Hogan was a particularly bad case. And I'd seen Sam Snead use his famous croquet-style putter to beat his yips. I decided to try a similar trick. I changed my grip, reversing my hands when I held a putter. And it worked … I won a tournament. Now I was convinced that it was not my attitude or technique. I had an affliction, and I was determined to conquer it. Yet the improvement with the changed grip was a honeymoon that did not last. I tried other tricks … putting cross-handed, and later changing the stance while putting so that I held the putter at an angle or even putted "side-saddle". I changed putters, going through longer and heavier ones, and then even the "pendulum". Every change worked for a short while, as if I had tricked my own mind into being normal. But the trickery was soon discovered and the problem came back … You are the first doctor I have consulted.

'Doc, I must say that I had some weird ideas as well. Someone suggested that perhaps the fault was in my selection of the golf balls. Of course, when you are putting, the aerodynamics of the ball should not matter, but how it moves on the green is important. You probably know that balls have compression ratings, and you match this with your stroke. A pro can advise you on that … nothing mysterious about it. There is also a number on the ball that indicates the number of dimples.'

'Oh, yes, the dimples! I've always wondered about the dimples – how are they determined? Do you actually count them, and does it matter?' I interrupted.

'You know that Haskell designed the first rubber-cored ball in the latter nineteenth century. Balls before that were made of, among other things, wood, goose feathers and horse hide, gutta etc. In the early twentieth century, Taylor applied the dimple pattern to the Haskell ball to give it better aerodynamics – it increased the lift and reduced the drag on the ball, helping it in the flight. Ever since then, we have had these dimpled balls. Who determines the number of dimples, I don't know. Perhaps there is some science behind it. Whenever I have looked at the number, it always seems to be even. I don't know why. The number of dimples is usually between 300 and 500. I read somewhere that the world record for the number of dimples is 1070, which included larger and smaller dimples. I thought – may be if I find a special ball, it will take my demons away. I hunted around and discovered that there was one ball on the market with odd-numbered dimples – exactly 333. Two of these made '666", and there – I thought this could be my answer – the magic I was waiting for.

'The first round I played with this "son of the devil" ball – as I called it – was a dream. No sign of the yips! It was totally irrational. I spoke to a friend about it, and he laughed. Was I going nuts? Thankfully, the yips returned in the very next round.'

'Thankfully?' I mused.

'You see, doc, it's ironical. I would have given anything in my possession to get rid of the yips. But would I give up my sanity? I don't believe in God, let alone the Devil. I run away from any superstitions. How could I make myself believe that the number of dimples could cure my yips? I would have fallen in my own eyes. I'd rather seek out a professional to find a cure.'

Faced with a problem about which I knew little, I sought refuge in that haven for the ignorant – the library. There was considerable lay literature on the yips, most of it amateurish, rather opinionated and somewhat emotive. Few great golfers were said to have escaped it. The Scottish-American golfer Tommy Armour (1894–1968), nicknamed the Silver Scot, is said to have popularised the term 'yips'. He temporarily lost his eyesight from a mustard gas explosion in World War I, only to regain the sight in his right eye. This did not prevent him from taking up golf and going on to win the US Open in 1927 and the British Open in 1931. In 1927, only a week after his US Open victory, he shot an 'archaeopteryx', an 18-over par on a 5-par hole at the Shawnee Open. This still stands as a record for the highest score on one hole in PGA history.[3]

Sam Snead, or 'Slammin' Sammy', was the most discussed of all the famous yippers. Snead is recognised as one of the golfing greats, having won six majors and 82 PGA tour events.

His advice to golfers was: 'Keep close count of your nickels and dimes, stay away from whiskey, and never concede a putt.' After having holed the course at St Andrews four times in 290 strokes in 1946 to fend off 225 challengers, this most graceful of golfers[4] was later so severely limited in his short putts that he chose to putt facing the hole with the ball between his feet. When this was outlawed, he developed his croquet-style or 'side-winding' technique in which he would stand, feet together, in a crouched position and hold the putter with an inverted left hand grip with 18 inches separating the hands. Unfortunately, this style too was quickly outlawed.

Bernhard Langer, the German golfer who was the inaugural World Number 1 when the official world golf rankings were introduced in 1986, battled with the yips for much of his career. While he played in ten Ryder Cups with five wins, he is best remembered for the missed 5-foot putt in the 1991 Ryder Cup that would have produced a tie and allowed the European team to retain the trophy. Other greats like Walter Hagen and Byron Nelson also fell victim to the yips.

The medical fraternity had largely ignored the yips. A rare exception was Jack Foster,[5] who in 1977 wrote a light-hearted article in *World Medicine*, making it clear that the yips had been grouped with the other 'occupational cramps (or palsies) (or neuroses)' and had been called golfer's cramp. No detailed description of the signs and symptoms of this disorder, if disorder it indeed was, existed. An important task then was to try to establish whether a particular set of signs and symptoms could be described that accurately defined this disorder; that is, to delineate the syndrome of golfer's cramp. This is often the first step in trying to establish a medical disorder, by providing coherence to the clinical presentation of the condition. I did this by inviting the participation of affected golfers in a research study.[6] Twenty golfers considered by themselves and their peers to be suffering from 'a bad case of the yips' agreed to be my guinea pigs. Now I had detailed anecdotes, and from these a fairly consistent picture of golfer's cramp emerged. While my own observations were under way, a study was published in the journal *Neurology* describing a survey of golfers with the yips by researchers from the University of California in Los Angeles.[7] Their findings agreed with my own. This heartened me, as *Neurology* is a highly respected medical journal and often sets the standard for the field.

The typical golfer with the yips in my study was a male in his late thirties who had been playing competitive golf since his teens. He had had no obvious technical problems with his game, often considered himself 'a very good putter' and played at a very low handicap. He first developed the problem in a stressful tournament when he experienced a sudden spasm or jerk in his forearm and/or hand muscles during the execution of short putts so that he was unable to control the stroke. The golfers I examined reported various kinds of disturbances, alone or in combination: the smooth movement of the stroke was overcome by a sudden, uncontrollable jerk; spasm of the hand and forearm muscles impaired smooth movement of the putter; and either the backward or the forward swing 'froze' and had to be brought to a jerky conclusion. These golfers also reported problems with the fixation of gaze on the ball. Most good golfers describe that when they attempt to putt, they can 'see' a line from the ball to the hole, and this is usually the direction the ball takes. The yips sufferers reported that they had stopped seeing that imaginary 'line'. The strokes affected were short putts (from 1 to 8 feet from the hole) and chips,[8] with the rest of the game being relatively unaffected. The problem recurred intermittently and started to generalise to other playing situations so that a fair number had problems even during practice sessions. It seemed that some deficit had developed in their ability to execute the finely controlled stroke of putting, but this deficit became apparent only when the mind was stressed. One golfer likened it to a scorpion lying curled in the recesses of the brain. The arousal of competition awakened it, and the sting in its tail was sharp and painful. It was also a capricious disorder, and could not always be predicted to occur, thus adding to the frustration it caused. There were periods when it would disappear, like a scorpion sleeping through winter, but in its case without any apparent reason. It would then strike again, and quite unexpectedly. Only one of my subjects reported complete recovery. The others continued to play in spite of the yips, although not at the same handicap. Most subjects had used 'trick' strategies to overcome the yips with at least partial success. These strategies included changing the putter (making it longer, or heavier, or reversed, or 'pendulum'), changing the grip (reversing hands, separating hands, cross-handed), changing the stance (putting 'side-saddle', changing head position, holding putter at an angle) and altering the point of gaze fixation at the time of the stroke.

As a general rule, all subjects were normal on examination physically and neurologically. Their fine coordination on testing was normal. Six out of 20 golfers, however, had gone on to develop coordination problems with one or more other fine movements such as writing, typing, or other sports such as tennis, ping pong and snooker, suggesting that they probably had a predisposition to this kind of disorder.

Having satisfied myself that the disorder had a definite pattern of presentation, which was reasonably similar from one golfer to another – and qualified for the status of a 'syndrome' in medical terms – the next task was to look at factors that predisposed any particular golfer to develop the yips. Was, as is generally believed, the yips all in the mind? Was it really a kind of neurosis that took a particular form in golfers? Was it a manifestation of anxiety that became particularly intense at the time of putting? The obvious strategy used to decide this question was to compare the affected golfers with a group of unaffected golfers who were similar in most respects except for the fact that they had never yipped.

Fortunately, I was able to attract 20 such golfers who were of the same age and golfing experience, and played at about the same handicap as the affected golfers would have if they did not have the yips. The two groups were compared on a number of measures of anxiety, depression, obsessionality and other psychiatric problems. No differences emerged on any of these measures. None of the study participants could be diagnosed as suffering from a psychiatric illness on examination. They did not emerge as more anxious, or depressed, or competitive, or 'neurotic' in general. I analysed the results further, dividing the affected golfers into two subgroups: 12 golfers who were severely affected and eight who were only mildly so. The severely affected golfers considered themselves more anxious than the others, but the two groups again did not differ appreciably on any of the measures used in the study. These findings were not what would be expected if the yips was a form of anxiety disorder or neurosis, thus giving the lie to the popular notion. Moreover, it is extremely unusual for a neurotic disorder to start in the late thirties, as was the case for golfer's cramp. This was not to say that anxiety (or, more correctly, arousal) did not have a role to play. It did seem to worsen the disorder, or bring about its manifestation in a particular situation, but it could not be said to be its cause.

In some ways this was a sad revelation. It gave the lie to some colourful psychological theories. Psychoanalysts have long thought that disorders of this kind represent an unconscious aggressive impulse that manifests itself in the form of a cramp, a kind of misdirection of aggression that really turns upon itself. Instead of being able to express his aggression normally, the individual tried to suppress it – a kind of unconscious control over the aggression. The control was not completely successful, and the aggression was not immediately obvious, even to the person himself. Not unlike many matters psychoanalytical, it was possibly sexual in origin. The masterful execution of long drives may be considered the epitome of masculinity, whereas the gracefulness of putting symbolised the feminine side of golf. All individuals have a masculine and a feminine side to their personality, and generally these are able to be reconciled satisfactorily. In a man, a revelation of the feminine side should not lead to alarm! In the yipper, a proper reconciliation of these two conflicting aspects does not occur. The putting is the feminine stroke of golf, characterised by its gentleness and curvaceous execution. No wonder the 'masculine' golfer falls to pieces at its feet. All the participants in my study were male, which is what one would have predicted from this theory. However, as seductive as this hypothesis is on the surface, it is entirely speculative, and not a shred of evidence has been presented to support it. I did not find my subjects any more aggressive or sexually confused than the average golfer, or indeed the average man. Incidentally, the problem is said to exist in female golfers as well. During the period of recruitment of participants for the study I did excite some interest in female golfers, but they did not come forth for an interview.

Despite his aggressive competitiveness on the green, Henry was a mild-mannered chap who waited patiently for me when I was running late, spoke with respect and never raised his voice. He bore no scars of schoolyard brawls, and was not known to throw his weight around in his school days. He had been popular with his peers and had kept his mates from his school days. He had no concerns about his masculinity either. A tall and handsome fellow, he had been popular with girls and had maintained a number of close relationships. Women liked his caring nature, and found him easy to talk to. It seemed to me that his Mars and Venus were well reconciled. He would have given little joy to the classical psychoanalyst.

A more common psychological explanation put forward for the 'yips' is that this disorder is a form of neurosis – a conversion disorder. The basis of this is anxiety, from whatever cause, that fails to find its normal expression and is 'converted' into a physical symptom, in this case a jerk or spasm. The mind is more comfortable in experiencing the anxiety in the form of a physical symptom rather than in its raw form as a mental phenomenon, as the theory goes. If this is true, the disorder should behave like a neurosis. It should occur in individuals prone to neurotic disorders: anxious, depressed or dependent individuals, who reveal a pattern of neurotic responses in their lives, who manifest 'neurosis' in most of life situations, and who deal with the disability in a 'neurotic' fashion. Neurotic individuals do not go through life plainly or effortlessly. Their emotions govern their existence. They react to happenings in their lives in an exaggerated manner and thereby cope poorly with stress. They need people to hold their hands. What should be a walk through the park can seem like a trek through a wood with hidden monsters. In colloquial terms, they suffer from 'acopia', an inability to handle what are relatively normal tribulations of human existence. My participants were none of these, but rather well-adjusted men who were otherwise successful in life.

Henry was one of them. He was a driven individual who could shrug off adversity with nary a scar. He thrived on competition and sought challenges. If he had any neurosis, it was his love of golf! He had made golf his life and his career, yet was prepared to give it up if he was told that his golfing career was over. He was willing to face life all over again, in a new guise bereft of green fields and flags and clubs. This was no 'neurotic man'!

If not a form of neurosis, what kind of disorder is golfer's cramp? One hypothesis is that golfer's cramp is the result of a disturbance in the part of the brain that controls finely coordinated movements. The most likely site for this problem is a mass of nerve cells lying deep in the brain and known as the basal ganglia. This 'biological' hypothesis is again speculative as no definite abnormality has been demonstrated in the basal ganglia, or indeed anywhere else in the brain, in any affected golfer. But a number of general observations point to this conclusion.

It is perhaps appropriate at this stage to draw an analogy with other occupational cramps, the best-known such disorder being writer's cramp. This disorder has been described in the medical literature since the early nineteenth century, but the first influential scientific paper on it was published by the great British neurologist Sir William Gowers in 1877.[9] Writer's cramp is now recognised to be common, and most doctors have seen one or more cases in their clinical practice. The first symptom described is a sense of stiffness of fingers after prolonged writing. This becomes progressively worse and results in a cramp of the thumb and index finger of the writing hand, resulting initially in a cramping of the writing and later making it impossible to write. The individual experiences no symptoms when he (or she) is not writing. The hand seems to work just fine. He can eat quite well using a fork and knife, shave with the affected hand and even play a musical instrument without difficulty. He has no problem in holding the pen appropriately. But the merest attempt to write can result in painful contraction of muscles and crude spontaneous movement that may rip the paper.

When this individual consults a neurologist, the news is both good and bad. The good news is that on examination, the nervous system is normal – the neurologist is unable to detect any signs of abnormality. He may even be sent for some laboratory tests used to detect neurological disease – measuring the conductivity of impulses in the nerves, or looking at the contractility of muscles. All of these turn out to be normal. The specialist's verdict – there is nothing wrong with you. Herein lies the bad news – the disorder is dismissed as being either trivial or 'psychological'. But does the lack of detectable abnormality equate with 'being normal'? Is the abnormality not in the fact that function has been affected? A hand that once could write effortlessly now goes into spasm at the slightest suggestion of the act. Surely that is not normal! The disability it produces is not merely someone's imagination.

For decades neurologists found it impossible to accept that writer's cramp could be a neurological disorder. Neurology has a proud tradition of being a rigorously scientific discipline based on astute observation and demonstrable abnormality. The discipline finds it difficult to cope with the subtle vagaries of the mind. Writer's cramp is too different from the usual abnormality seen in the clinic. Here is an individual who for all practical purposes is completely normal. On examination, his hand is normal. His muscles have good strength. He can manipulate his fingers with great dexterity for most tasks. He, in fact, has no complaints until he starts to write. The understandable reaction – this must be 'psychiatric'. This conclusion is supported by the observation that anxiety seems to make matters worse and, at least initially, sufferers report problems only when someone is watching them write. They often find ways of dealing with this problem by 'tricking their hand', as one sufferer put it. He initially switched to a thicker pen, and the problem was overcome but only for a few weeks. He then tried a different grip – from a pincer to a dagger-like grip. This again worked, but for some reason the relief was again temporary. He next switched to typing, and for several months there was no difficulty in manipulating the keyboard. In reality, he was not tricking the hand, but was somehow bypassing the dysfunctional system in the brain. In other words, the 'trick' worked in the brain region that controlled the complex movement of handwriting.

There is some evidence that we do develop patterns or 'motor plans' in the brain that guide complex movements. Writing is an activity that engages many muscles of the hand and arm with extreme precision. When a child begins to write, she takes one step at a time – each letter is an effort and the flow from one to another takes many months of practice. An adult writes without deliberation or effort. It is as if the brain has formed a routine that can operate almost automatically. That this routine is in the brain is evident from the fact that the muscles involved in the act of writing can be changed without much difficulty. We can switch from writing on a piece of paper with a pen to writing on a blackboard with chalk without thinking about it, and our handwriting does not change in the process. My signature on paper looks exactly like it does on a blackboard, yet the muscles I use to write on paper are quite different from those used to write on the board. It must be the constancy of the program in the brain that permits this switch to occur. The speculation therefore is that it must be some defect in this program that leads to writer's cramp by sending signals to the wrong muscles when the individual decides to write. By changing the grip, the program can be rebooted, so to speak, for some time. Writer's cramp usually affects individuals who write for a living, such as shorthand typists, stenographers, etc.[10] It is possibly related to some form of overuse, perhaps under stress. The abnormality is in the 'software program' of the brain whereas the neurologist is seeking a deficit in the hardware. This is what Sir David Marsden, a prominent neurologist from the National Hospital in Queen Square, London, tried to argue, but even his eminent position in the field was insufficient to convince the sceptical neurologists. It was only when he showed that some of the individuals with writer's cramp went on to develop dystonia, a disorder in which muscles of a body region (in this case the hand) contracted involuntarily, that they started to come around to his way of thinking. He also showed that some of the sufferers had a family history of dystonia. Some novel investigations, using special techniques, have demonstrated neurophysiological abnormalities in patients with writer's cramp, again supporting a neurological basis.

As we can see, writer's cramp is the perfect clinical analogy for the yips. It affects a well-practised and highly skilled movement, other fine movements are spared, and there are no obvious abnormalities on neurological examination. Similar disorders have been described in scores of other occupations. Musicians such as violinists and pianists are known to develop cramps in their fingers related to their craft. Similar problems have been described in typists, telegraphists, painters, sports people (snooker players, dart throwers, cricketers), bank tellers, cotton-twisters, cigar-rollers, knife-grinders, and barbers. The hands are parts of the body most frequently involved, presumably because it is with our hands that we perform skilled acts most often. But it is the skilled act that is dysfunctional and not the hand! And if other parts are involved in equally skilled activities, they too may become affected. The feet may get affected in ballerinas, and an affliction of the tongue has been described in a trombone player. Writer's cramp has been most extensively written about. Most investigators in this field now recognise writer's cramp, and by analogy other such disorders, as focal task-specific dystonias. As can be seen from my examination of 20 sufferers, golfer's cramp fits the same general description.

If it is indeed a dystonia that manifests itself only in one particular action (although occasionally spreading to other actions), what is its mechanism of development? This remains speculative. One suggestion is that the prolonged practice of the golf swing results in the formation of a 'motor plan' in the basal ganglia so that the movement can be carried out relatively automatically, much like the act of writing. This motor plan consists of a number of 'motor programs', which, like computer routines, are arranged in a hierarchic order. The programs are fairly stereotyped but not rigid. They are flexible enough to be slightly altered by input from the sensory organs, which is important since the golfing stroke must vary depending upon the distance from the hole, the nature of the putting green, the presence of any unevenness or moisture on the surface, and other such considerations. The motor program should also be modifiable by input from the higher centres of the brain, which have evaluated the information concerning wind speed and direction, humidity and such like. The motor plan then sends impulses to all the right muscles to contract or relax as the case may be in order to execute the stroke. In the case of the yips, this message somehow gets scrambled so that the wrong muscles contract, or contract to the wrong degree.

Do we know what disrupts this motor plan? No. It is possible that some individuals have a constitutional predisposition to a disturbance of the neurochemicals that are involved in the motor programs. We do know that a change does occur in neurochemistry of the basal ganglia with age, starting at 15 and reaching its peak effect in the thirties. We know that stress and anxiety lead to changes in the same brain chemicals. The increased workload that hundreds of hours of practice places on the brain cells may also be relevant. It is therefore not surprising that anxiety can stress the system until it becomes quite dysfunctional. We now have newer techniques of brain imaging that may be able to test this hypothesis by measuring the activity of brain cells while the individual is performing specific tasks. It is important to recognise that it is the most complex and well-mastered motor act that gets affected; in the case of golf, it is putting. Perhaps the complexity of the motor program makes it more vulnerable to abnormality. It is the most highly evolved conductor that falls prey to the affliction.

Meanwhile, what does this newer thinking on the yips offer to countless sufferers? There are no medicines that will cure their condition. The alleviation of anxiety and stress will have a mitigating effect, but again it is not a cure. A more important corollary is that remedial action at the very onset of the problem may be far more important than efforts at a later stage, as stress reduction or temporary cessation of golf play at that point may well arrest the condition at its onset. It may be advisable for golfers not to deny the problem in its early stages. 'It can't happen to me' is not true. It is certainly not a sign of psychiatric disturbance or mental weakness, and it is not an end to many more years of pleasurable golf.

And what of Henry? After only two sessions, he was beginning to appreciate the likely brain mechanisms behind his affliction. It led to a mixture of relief and disappointment. The realisation that you are a victim of your circumstances, or nature itself, might bring out anger in some people, but for Henry, it was fate's iron fist wrapped in the velvet glove that was his talent in golf. He was not one to pity himself. The disappointment was largely due to the fact that this had happened before his professional career had taken off. He could have lived with a Ben Hogan or a Sam Snead scenario, with the yips coming after a taste of success. Indeed, he would have been happy with lesser heights!

I decided to see him regularly to help him through this phase of indecision. He initially pressed me for treatment. There was no scientific evidence to guide me, but I knew that as a clinician, my strategies should be geared towards healing despite the lack of evidence. I mulled over this for a few days. If Henry had a life-threatening illness, I would have downplayed my ignorance and presented him with hope – a healer has no other road to take. I would even have nudged him to try experimental treatments. The nature of his disorder was such that I could not bring myself to hide the facts from him – I lay all the cards on the table. I offered him the choice of trying medicines. There are some drugs that sometimes work for dystonias, but I cautioned him that all of them had noticeable side effects, and drugs are generally known to fail in task-specific dystonias. These medicines are no more than blunt weapons, akin to using a hammer to fine tune a circuit. The drugs will go wherever the blood supply will take them, unable to restrict their actions to any specific brain region that may be malfunctioning. Moreover, without knowing the exact cause of the problem, a specific drug was not on the horizon. Henry was unwilling to even entertain the thought of using these drugs.

Another medication-based strategy was to try an anti-anxiety drug. There was an obvious problem here. I had told him that this was not an anxiety disorder – how could I then justify recommending an anti-anxiety drug? Moreover, the drugs generally used to treat increased anxiety, such as diazepam (Valium), were not only habituating, they were also likely to adversely affect his golf, and if they led to any improvement, it was likely to be temporary.

The other strategy was to use a drug some individuals use for social anxiety or stage fright, the so-called beta-blockers. Propranolol is the best-known of these drugs. The principle is simple: an anxiety-provoking situation leads to an increase in heart rate, which makes anxiety worse by means of a feedback mechanism. Propranolol slows the heart rate and thereby blocks this feedback and reduces anxiety. It thereby steadies the nerves in anxious individuals, but must be taken immediately before the event. Henry tried this on two occasions in a state tournament, and found himself to be steadier. It failed as a test for his yips as he did not experience any yips during this tournament. He was tormented by the fact that this might be construed as cheating. Most golf tournaments had not introduced drug testing, but there was much talk of the PGA tour introducing it. There was, in any case, a code of honour, and beta-blockers were treated with suspicion. In fact, some golfers who suffered from high blood pressure, a medical indication for the use of beta-blockers, had been switched to alternative treatments. Henry was unwilling to go down this path.

The only path open to Henry was to retrain his brain. This was a slow process that demanded patience and dedication. He would need to stop playing for some months, then start from the very basics. This strategy sometimes worked with writer's cramp. He would need the help of a professional coach. I had to refer him to someone who understood the golfing brain without ever having read neuroscience. I reluctantly bid him farewell. He had a few months to decide which direction he would take.

I met Henry two years later. He had decided not to become a professional golfer after all. He had gone back to university and was training to become a physiotherapist. He continued to play golf and got a lot of enjoyment from his game.

2

Shaking hands with Dr Strangelove

Who is it that can tell me who I am?

William Shakespeare, *King Lear* (1605–06)

… the cutting of this connecting tissue between the two hemispheres of the brain can be viewed as the ultimate symbolic act of Pisces, the Age of Polarities. It gives credence to the idea that the Day World can be separated from the Night World, and that rational functioning can be separated from intuitive functioning, and that masculine consciousness can be separated from feminine consciousness …

June Singer, *Androgyny*[1]

Robert was 20 years old when he came to our clinic. He presented as a rather prosaic individual, with a face bereft of emotion. His bowed head and stooped shoulders conveyed a sense of burden that I could not easily empathise with. The only word he had to say about himself was that he was 'epileptic'. Ordinarily, I would dismiss such an adjective as a dehumanising epithet, unworthy of a doctor's clinic. 'You suffer from epilepsy … are perhaps even consumed by it, but please do not call yourself epileptic,' I was beginning to reflect. If he was wearing the illness like a garment to wrap and conceal, then it was my job to unravel it layer by layer to reveal the person who lay within. But Robert's appellation was curiously apt!

His life was his epilepsy, and had always been so. He had epilepsy even before his earliest memories took him to the playful years of childhood. He had grown up with 'Oh, the poor kid's epileptic!' as he watched other children swim and ride bicycles and do all manner of 'hazardous' things. When the football coach agreed to have him practice with the other children, he had a seizure and was sent away for good. On his first date, the 'turn' scared the girl so much that word quickly got around about this 'complete whacko' who just stared and made queer noises while the frightened girl thought of a quick way to escape. The experience was enough for him to decide on celibacy and the life of a recluse. If he had been bright, he might have excelled at something that would have perhaps provided him with another defining activity. This was not to be, and when he visited me, the uppermost thought in his mind was 'If only I did not have epilepsy'. For this young man, life would begin after his last epileptic seizure. Many neurologists had attempted to give him that start in life and had failed.

An epileptic seizure is an electrical storm in the brain that overwhelms brain activity for a few moments, and may produce a convulsion or altered behaviour with usually a distinct lack of awareness for that period. Electrical signals are the natural modality of discourse in the brain, with neuronal activity being propagated by charged particles. In a normally functioning brain, this activity is highly regulated in order to process complex information. In epilepsy, an area in the brain, usually referred to as the 'epileptic focus', generates electrical signals with an autonomy and ferocity that sees these signals propagated through major regions of the brain, disrupting their normal activity and producing, in most cases, an alteration in consciousness and an abnormality in behaviour. In some cases, this leads to repetitive movements of the body, referred to as a convulsion, as happened occasionally to Robert. More frequently, however, his seizures resulted in a sudden loss of consciousness and a fall to the ground due to a loss of tone in the muscles that keep us upright. Bruises on his forehead were testimony to the frequent occurrence of these 'atonic' seizures in recent days.

A person with epilepsy experiences the full impact of a sudden loss of control over his actions, feelings and thoughts. It is literally a taking over … a kind of invasion of the mind by an alien force that ironically has arisen from within. It is not surprising that since antiquity, epilepsy has been regarded as a visitation by an outside spirit, malevolent in intent and totally powerful because of its startling suddenness. The individual, usually confident of his ability to exercise his free will, and secure in his autonomy, is powerless in the face of this turbulence. Should we not conceptualise human will as some orderly activity in the brain that is overwhelmed by a sudden electrical storm? This activity must furthermore be electromagnetic in its property in order to be so influenced. The subsequent course that Robert's condition took provided an interesting lesson in the neurobiology of free will.

It is fortunate that most epilepsy can be controlled by antiepileptic drugs that provide a brake on the genesis or propagation of the electrical storm. Robert's neurologists had applied their collective skills in finding the best combinations of drugs to treat his epilepsy, but to no avail. The drugs had conspired to reduce his alertness, and he had spent many years of schooling seemingly in a daze. He had emerged semiliterate, poorly equipped to obtain any marketable skills, bereft of friends, with but one characteristic – that of his epilepsy – providing the basis of his being. Robert was not someone to give up, however, and he sought a surgeon who could excise, and thus exorcise, the demon in his brain. He wanted my help to find this surgeon.

Removing a part of the brain that repeatedly produces epileptic discharges is a medically established procedure to cure epilepsy that does not respond to drug treatment. The prime requirement is the demonstration that most, if not all, seizures in that individual arise from a localisable focus in the brain. This brain region should then be, for most practical purposes, expendable. In other words, the surgeon should be able to remove it without producing substantive impairment in functional capacities. The preliminary investigations revealed that Robert's problem was not such that would easily lend itself to control with surgery. There was no one clear-cut focus of origin of his seizures, and his epilepsy possibly arose from multiple foci – there were many sparks that lit the fires in his brain. Surgery to remove one focus is doomed to fail in such cases, much like blocking one hole of a sieve to enable it to hold water.

While presenting this grim prognosis to him, I offered a ray of hope. A property of his epilepsy, particularly the atonic seizures, was that the full manifestation of the seizures occurred when the electrical discharge in the brain had spread to both hemispheres after having originated in one. There was a kind of surgery that could still be done that would not cure his epilepsy but could possibly provide him with much relief. If a surgeon was to operate to cut the connections between the two halves of the brain, thus interrupting the spread of the epileptic activity from one cerebral hemisphere to the other, the epilepsy, while not losing its bite, would renounce its viciousness. He would still have epileptic discharges but, because their path of spread in the brain was now blocked, he would no longer fall suddenly because of them, a prospect he found quite exciting. The operation I was referring to is called a corpus callosotomy – in simple terms, a splitting of the brain.

The human brain comprises two hemispheres, with the left hemisphere controlling the right side of the body and vice versa. The two hemispheres communicate with each other through a big body (corpus callosum) that lies in the middle, consisting of more than 200 million fibres that cross over and provide a unity to the brain. It never ceases to amaze me that all these fibres can be cut and the individual, for all practical purposes, continues to behave and perform normally.[2] This very fact offered Robert some hope for which he was grateful. After a week of investigations in our ward to confirm the nature of his epilepsy and consider his suitability for surgery, he was handed over to the neurosurgeon for a complete corpus callosum section.

I next saw him three days after his surgery. He had recovered from the acute effects of the operation, and was fully conscious. He told me that when he first tried to get out of bed, he found his left leg to be 'lazy', and he had some problem in walking, having to drag the leg. This was obviously mild weakness of the leg, which lasted only a few hours. He now felt that all his limbs were in good working order. It was too early to say whether the surgery had produced a worthwhile gain in his epilepsy. He had not experienced a seizure since the surgery, but this could have been due to the many drugs administered during and after the anaesthesia.

After having spoken to him, I walked over to the nurses' station in the ward. As soon as she saw me peering into Robert's chart, an excited nurse came over to tell me about this 'strange episode' she had witnessed. She had offered Robert a cup of tea which he accepted with his right hand, but as he was about to take it to his lips, the left hand groped his right wrist so tightly that the tea spilt all over him. The left hand still did not let go, and she had to help Robert disentangle the two hands. 'It was as if the left hand did not belong to Robert at all. An alien spirit had taken over the control of his left hand,' the nurse remarked. I was nonplussed. Had I missed something in my brief examination of Robert? I returned to do a more complete examination.

I found Robert to be in good spirits. He said that he was pleased to see me again, and surprised that I had come back so soon. I performed a full neurological examination on him. His left arm and leg were a bit clumsy, but the muscle strength in the limbs was normal. He tended to hold his left arm hanging limply on the side, but this was because he 'preferred to do most things with the right', as he put it. It did seem that the arm movements were flowing more easily on the right side, and the left arm was being used sparingly. Robert was, however, not aware of any difference. I asked him to copy a tapping rhythm with his left hand to test his ability to do repetitive movements, and he had no difficulty in doing so. I also wanted to find out whether some of the high-level sensory functions were preserved in both hands. One of these functions is to be able to identify objects just by touching and feeling them. With his eyes closed, he could identify some coins placed one by one in his right hand, but could not identify them when placed in the left. This disturbance has previously been called 'astereognosis' and reflects the brain's inability to recognise an object when information from touching the object is available to the brain. The explanation for this lay in the fact that the ability to recognise and put a name to an object lies in the left hemisphere. The sensory information from his left hand was being conveyed to the right hemisphere, but because of the cut in the corpus callosum, this could not travel to the left for the recognition to occur. I next asked him to write his name, first with the left, even though I knew he was right-handed. He produced an illegible doodle. Normally, right-handed individuals are, with some effort, able to produce legible, albeit poorly formed writing with the left hand – Robert had lost this ability. He was aware of the poor effort of his left hand and offered an excuse: 'My left hand is having some difficulty today – maybe it is too soon after the surgery.' The real reason was that the message to write the name had to travel from the left to the right hemisphere, and the road had been blocked.

I then asked him to write his name with the other hand – and I was not prepared for what I saw! When he began to write with the right hand, the left came and pushed his right hand such that the pen tore through the page. I had to help him loosen the grip of the left hand for him to continue. I next gave him a plastic cup filled with water to drink with his right hand. As he picked it up, the left hand groped about, then came and crushed the cup, spilling the water on the bed. He gazed at me with a confused look on his face. He was clearly nonplussed by this behaviour of his left hand.

'I don't know what is happening to me,' he said.

'Can you not control its movements?' I asked him.

'It has a mind of its own … I know that it is my own hand, but it is not acting under my command.'

Robert could not understand what was happening to him. He was aware of the bizarre nature of what had happened, and seemed to be frightened by it. He went so far as to ask me. 'Do you think I am going crazy, Dr Sachdev?'

'It is indeed a strange sight, and not easy to explain, but it is most definitely not a sign of madness. We think it can all be explained on the basis of the surgery you had.'

Robert was further distressed as the hand groped around, tugging at his shirt as he tried to hold it with his right hand. He was looking toward me for reassurance. I hesitated to offer it. I had read about this symptom after corpus callosotomy but had never seen a case before. I offered him some words of reassurance, suggesting that this problem was likely to be temporary and would pass. I did not know enough about the problem to sound completely convincing. Thoughts were welling up in my mind. Would he ever be completely normal again? Would the two sides of the brain, which had been deliberately separated, be able to communicate once again? Had we inadvertently created two Roberts? Would the wholeness of Robert be restored? I made my way straight to the library.

A patient whose left hand behaved in the manner I had witnessed was first described by Kurt Goldstein, a pioneering German neurologist and psychiatrist, in 1908.[3] Goldstein had a holistic view of the human being, and formed his opinions on human nature on the basis of his studies of brain injuries. His best-known work is *The Organism*, which was published in English in 1995. The patient of interest to us was a 57-year-old woman whose left hand grabbed her throat and almost choked her. His patient had multiple lesions in the brain involving the right hemisphere and the corpus callosum. As he wrote:

> On one occasion the hand grabbed her own neck and tried to throttle her, and could only be pulled off by force. Similarly, it tore off the bedcovers against the patient's will ... She soon was complaining about her hand; that it is a law unto itself, an organ without will; when once it has got hold of something, it refuses to let go: ... 'I suppose there must be an evil spirit in it.'[4]

It was Dr A. I. Akelaitis, an American psychiatrist, who first described the syndrome after corpus callosotomy performed for epilepsy in 1945.[5] Since then, many such cases have been reported in the literature.[6] The term 'alien hand' had its origin in the French descriptor 'Le signe de la main étrangère' of Brion and Jedynak in 1972,[7] two Frenchmen who described patients with tumours of the corpus callosum, who were unable to recognise the left hand as their own when touched by the right hand with their eyes closed. These authors did not refer to involuntary or uncontrollable movements in their descriptions. The current conceptualisation of the alien hand is after Joseph Bogen[8] of the University of Southern California in Los

Angeles, who in 1979 described the involuntary behaviour of the left hand in the split-brain patient as its main feature.

Robert's left hand is also reminiscent of the antics of the mad scientist Dr Strangelove in the Stanley Kubric 1964 black satirical movie by the same name. Dr Strangelove was a former Nazi physicist who becomes adviser to the American President Muffley in the movie, and translates his German name 'Merk-würdigliebe' to its English equivalent. Peter Sellers, who played this role in the movie, wears a black glove on his right hand, which behaves in an anarchic manner – twice making the Heil Hitler salute to the President and once trying to strangle Dr Strangelove himself.

It is remarkable that Robert recognised the hand as being his own, but one that moved of its own 'volition' and interfered with the activity of the other hand. This is the feature that made Della Sala, Marchetti and Spinnler,[9] from the San Paolo Hospital in Milan, Italy refer to it as the 'anarchic' rather than the alien hand, but Geschwind and his colleagues[10] from the University of California at Los Angeles had a patient who felt that 'someone from the moon' was controlling her hand.

The experience you have when a part of your body that was previously fully in your control but now moves with autonomy, and generally to no purpose, can be very disconcerting indeed. The frantic attempts that Robert made to control the movements of his left hand were a statement of the agony he suffered at his peculiar fate. If he had lost awareness of his hand – or indeed the very knowledge that it was his own – he might have been less distressed by it. He could now do little more than be astonished by the antics of his left hand. While he could still use his hand, he had to focus on it, look at it

constantly and deal with its 'laziness'. Once, while performing the finger-nose test in which I asked him to touch his
nose, his left pointer entered his mouth. 'I wonder why it did
that,' Robert remarked. 'Stupid left hand!' This critical appreciation of the actions of the anarchic hand were referred to as
'l'autocritique interhémispherique' by French neurologists,[11]
painting the interesting image of one hemisphere criticising
the other for bad etiquette.

Robert's left hand was not always a clumsy automaton. At
times, it showed a remarkable uncanniness in annoying him.
While I was interviewing him, the phone rang. I saw Robert
pick the receiver with the right hand to answer the call, but
the left hand rose quickly and attempted to hang up the phone.
He tried to slap his left hand with the right, and dropped the
receiver in the process. The phone rang again, and I witnessed
a repetition of this child-like conflict. Both hands were being
activated, one purposefully, the other with a strange 'purpose'
of senseless interference. The nurse had observed a similar
scene in another setting. His right hand was seen buttoning
up his shirt while the left went behind it unfastening those
very buttons. Both hands belonged to Robert. He was not in
two minds about his actions; he was clear about wanting to
answer the phone and buttoning up. Which one was carrying
out Robert's 'real' instructions? For him, the right hand was
the one controlled by his will. There was no ambivalence that
he ostensibly harboured.[12] The conflict was between the hands,
not one that he experienced in his mind. In fact, he was critical
of his left hand in that it would not do his bidding.[13]

I asked him if it felt like being two people in one body. I
remember his response quite vividly: 'I feel like one person all

right, not two. It is this hand that has a mind of its own ... as if it is no longer part of me ... like an appendage with a different control ... But ... I know it is my hand.'

The strange behaviour of Robert's left hand takes one on a long journey of the concept of the double-brain[14] that began in its rudimentary form with the philosopher René Descartes (1596–1650) and reached its zenith in the debates of the classical neurologists of the nineteenth century. Anatomists were understandably struck by the duality of the hemispheres of the brain and the large size, central location and widespread connections of the corpus callosum. Thomas Willis, the famous neuroanatomist of the seventeenth century, was one of many who considered it to be the likely seat of the soul. When it became clear that brain regions had specialised functions, with the left hemisphere being the basis of language, the concept of the corpus callosum as a two-way traffic channel became current. Its existence, in some way, provided unity to a bicameral mind. Its status had been down-graded to that of a bridge, and the question being asked by many scientists was: what if this bridge is destroyed? Does it lead to a person having two minds, or is it that only one mind results but the presence of the unconscious becomes apparent? If there are two minds, is one dominant over the other? Does it also lead to two selves? Not surprisingly, physicians were tempted into amateur philosophy as philosophers still had developed little interest in the actual workings of the brain.

The double-brain theory was a potent source of psycho-logical theorising in the nineteenth century, some of which was the consequence of over-enthusiastic leaps of logic. An interesting concept put forward by Frederic Myers, one of the founders of the British Society for Psychical Research, was that of the subliminal self. Myers wanted to develop a theory of the subconscious mind because he believed, like many others of his time, that everyday consciousness represented only a fraction of the total self. This subliminal self, he argued, came from the right side of the brain.[15] To support his ideas, he cited the report by the Reverend P. H. Newham, who had observed individuals producing automatic writing using a planchette, the forerunner of the ouija or spirit board used to communicate with spirits.[16] He drew attention to the 'low moral character' of the personality that emerged in the course of the automatic writing. He attributed this to the fact that this was the product of the right half of the brain, a part that was undisciplined and untrained because it was not habitually used during everyday actions. To further support the argument, Myers cited the frequent presence of errors in the writing produced by the planchette board – words written backwards, transposed, in mirror-image or distorted – that reminded him of the errors of aphasic patients who had suffered damage to the left cerebral hemisphere and were arguably using their right lobes.[17]

Other physicians, who did not delve into the paranormal, also presented cases to argue for a different 'personality' for the two hemispheres, and a division of consciousness because of dissociation between the two. The case of Louis Vivé reported by two French physicians, Bourru and Burot,[18] was an interesting example. He was a young man who, after a turbulent childhood, developed hysterical symptoms at the age of 14 years after narrowly escaping being bitten by a viper. He developed paralysis and anaesthesia in different parts of the body. When Bourru and Burot saw him, he had paralysis and anaesthesia in the right side of the body, suggesting an abnormality of the left cerebral hemisphere. The personality characteristics were striking: he was noted to be insolent, impulsive and uninhibited. He would 'harangue the hospital staff with monkey-like impudence, preach radicalism in politics and atheism in religion, try to fondle people who pleased him and behave in a violent, greedy and quarrelsome manner'.[19] With the aid of magnets and metals,[20] his hemiplegia (weakness of one half of the body) and hemianaesthesia (loss of sensation on one side of the body) was transferred to the right side of his body, and a remarkable transformation occurred in his personality. From being a 'savage', he was transformed into a gentleman, who spoke clearly and respectfully and was diplomatic in his comments on religion and politics. Other manipulations resulted in variations of his symptoms as well as his personality to forms intermediate between the extreme 'right' and 'left'.[21] Louis had become a messenger for an independent right-brain consciousness, crude though it was considered to be.

Another case that attracted much attention in the late nineteenth century was the 'Welsh' case of Dr Lewis Bruce, a Scottish physician.[22] This patient alternated between being right- and left-handed. When right-handed, he spoke fluent English and could understand and converse in Welsh. He also was 'restless, destructive, thievish, and [is] constantly playing practical jokes on his fellow patients. He exhibits a fair amount of intelligence … His memory is, however, a blank to anything that occurred during the Welsh stage …' When left-handed, he spoke in Welsh but this was unintelligible to other Welsh-speaking patients. He appeared to have no comprehension of English. He was shy, suspicious and underactive. Bruce argued strongly for a duality of the brain, but was uncertain as to what he should attribute the apparent 'dementia' of the right hemisphere – a product of madness or of poor development? The idea had become prevalent that the left hemisphere was the educated and 'civilised' part of the brain whereas the right was the untamed, raw, emotive, indeed the 'vulgar' part. Automatic writing, attributed to the right hemisphere by Myers, often included swear words, although the fact that this was still language was conveniently ignored.

The double brain hypothesis continued into the early part of the twentieth century but its critics had gradually become more vocal. Eugen Bleuler,[23] the famous Swiss psychiatrist who coined the term 'schizophrenia', reported a remarkable case of unilateral (one-sided) delirium. The patient suffered from general paralysis of the insane, a form of tertiary syphilis, and was admitted to the psychiatric hospital in Zurich. He was relaxed on the left side of his body, but his right side was in a state of marked agitation. The right hand would seize and pull things, grab at ropes, chop things with an axe and sling away dramatically, and while all this restless activity occurred, the patient could use language normally. The left hand behaved in a civilised manner, readjusting the bedclothes and wiping the patient's mouth, but during its activity, the patient's speech was greatly limited. Bleuler considered this to be evidence that an individual's personality could be sustained by one hemisphere. Indeed, cases have been described in which the individual has one functioning hemisphere, either because of abnormal brain development or hemispherectomy (surgical removal of one hemisphere, usually due to severe epilepsy) or infarction (neuronal death due to the interruption of blood supply to the hemisphere), with little clinical impairment evident on superficial examination.

Extraordinary as the above cases were, the concept of brain duality was challenged by many investigators, not the least because hypnotic phenomena were prevalent equally on both sides of the body. The dual brain theorists had carried their claims too far in order to explain every discrepancy in the mind. As Pierre Janet, the famous French psychiatrist known for his theories of hysteria that preceded Sigmund Freud, put it, 'In fact, we have, all of us, two brains, and we are neither madmen, nor somnambulists, nor mediums.'[24] It is useful to point out that the unconscious processing of information was not being questioned, but rather the theory that the two halves of the brain had independent functioning – indeed personalities – and that it was their imbalance that led to psychiatric symptomatology. There were alternative, and more acceptable, explanations for the cases described above, and early in the twentieth century, the focus had moved on to these. The idea that the brain was but a diffuse mass of cells that mysteriously produced various cognitions was not tenable. Specialisation of different brain regions was well accepted by then, especially the understanding that language function was the domain of the left hemisphere and our ability to navigate spatially and construct 2D and 3D figures that of the right hemisphere.

The role of the corpus callosum as a conduit for the interhemispheric transfer of information was brought home by the work of a German neurologist, Hugo Liepmann.[25] Liepmann, a professor of neurology at the University of Berlin, was a former student of the famous neurologist Carl Wernicke who instilled in him the desire to localise cognitive processes in specific brain regions. Wernicke is of course well known to all medical students for his pioneering work on the localisation of human speech to the left hemisphere in what is called Wernicke's area. Liepmann described a patient who, on initial examination, seemed to have lost the ability to comprehend language or to make sense of objects in his environment. The patient attempted to use his right hand to perform a task, but was obviously unsuccessful. He held his left hand inactive by his side, even though it was not paralysed. When ordered to use his left hand, while his right hand was restrained, the man demonstrated an ability to carry out basic commands,[26] suggesting that his comprehension was not defective but that he was unable to carry out a complex action with his right hand, a phenomenon Liepmann called apraxia.[27] The realisation that an individual could lose the ability to perform a motor task when the hand was not paralysed and the command was being understood was a novel concept at that time. Liepmann argued that the stroke had affected the left parietal lobe, which was responsible for converting the intention of performing an act into its actual performance through the execution of a motor program. The right hemisphere was still able to do so, thereby explaining the ability of the left hand to perform these tasks. But why could the right hemisphere not compensate for the incapacity of its left twin? The likely explanation was that in addition to the parietal lobe, the corpus callosum had also been affected by the stroke. This bold argument was proven to be correct after the patient's death when the pathologist who did an autopsy on the brain did indeed demonstrate lesions in both regions.[28]

Liepmann's ideas were consistent with the localisationistic (brain functions were localised to certain brain regions) and connectionistic (brain regions were connected to other brain regions through axons) views of the brain that Wernicke had expounded. Liepmann's view of the corpus callosum was further supported by the case described by Kurt Goldstein that I mentioned at the beginning of this chapter. The debate about the nature of these phenomena continued for the next half century. It was in the 1960s that systematic studies about the neuropsychological functions subserved by the two cerebral hemispheres were conducted by neuroscientists like Roger Sperry, Michael Gazzaniga and a string of their followers at the California Institute of Technology in San Francisco. Sperry went on to share the 1980 Nobel Prize for Medicine with two other pioneering neuroscientists, David Hubel and Torsten Wiesel. Sperry tested ten patients who had undergone a section of the corpus callosum for epilepsy, and concluded that each half of the brain contained consciousness. To quote him: 'Each hemisphere is indeed a conscious system in its own right, perceiving, thinking, remembering, reasoning, willing, and emoting, all at a characteristically human level, and ... both the left and the right hemisphere may be conscious simultaneously in different, even in mutually conflicting, mental experiences that run along in parallel.'[29]

Scientists continued to speak about the dominant (or major) and non-dominant (or minor) hemispheres, but it became evident that the so-called minor hemisphere was able to produce emotional responses and influence behaviour independently of the left hemisphere without the individual acknowledging verbally that he or she was aware of these responses. Was there indeed a double consciousness or a duality of mind after all? Or was it more fruitful to conceptualise it in terms of specialisation in the brain, with the coordinated activity in these regions laying the foundation for an individual's personality and consciousness? Was the right/left difference the basis for the two dichotomies of existence: rational and emotive–intuitive, propositional and appositional, yin and yang, science and art? The debates that followed were fertile ground for a range of ideas on politics, culture, society, arts and philosophy,[30] which I will not discuss here.

The above was a brief historical detour to flesh out the background to Robert's experience of an anarchic hand. What the activities of the hand were telling us was that the left hemisphere was normally responsible for a coordinated manual response to verbal stimuli, either external commands or self-injunctions. The right hemisphere could, nevertheless, move the left hand in response to emotional stimuli, but this activity appeared to be out of the person's volitional control. Does this mean that the will of an individual is dependent upon language? Or is it merely the communication of the will that is at fault, so that the right hemisphere is unable to communicate the intactness of the will to the left hemisphere if the two have been disconnected? To put it simply, the right hand could communicate with the person and the observer while the left was condemned to silence (internal and external) because of its lack of language. Is it arguable then that human will is localisable in the brain, is closely linked to the centres that process language, and is in fact in the left half of the brain?

This is not such a strange proposition as it may seem on the surface!

Human volition has two aspects to it: the awareness to an observer that an individual is the 'doer' of an action, and to that individual that he or she (the 'I') is responsible for the action. Imagine a situation where you are the only person in the universe. Imagine that you are Adam before Eve was created. Would the concept of your will, in contrast with another's will, still have meaning? It is possible that you may still have a concept of I-ness and fear that alien spirits may take that away. The context of the other person – the fact that we live and deal with other people throughout our lives – assumes a communicability of the will and therefore a dependence on language. The concept of the self must engage a part of the brain – probably the prefrontal cortex in the front of the brain – that can initiate the act, observe it and reiterate its origin from the 'self'. It is possible that the development of this feedback system was in the left side of the brain owing to its specialisation for language. Robert was not only stating that the left hand was not in his control; he also expressed surprise at its actions, which he was unable to curb through internally generated injunctions. The right hand did not suffer the same fate, even though the corpus callosum is a two-way street and therefore the left hemisphere had suffered the same disconnection as the right.

Let me remind the reader that we are attributing only one aspect of I-ness to the left hemisphere: the fact of having performed a volitional motor act. The same may not be true for the I-ness of an emotion or a musical tune or an image. The idea of a will to imagine or feel may well be in the right hemisphere, but its expression would still hinge on its communication to the language centres of the brain. But, hold on! Perhaps this entire thinking is a bit warped and the issue of localisation in the brain has been taken too far. A brain region does not generate an idea, or an act, or an emotion – let alone a person – in isolation. It is networked with other brain regions that in turn link with other regions. It is possibly the coming together of activation of a set of interconnected brain regions that creates the neurobiological basis of the realisation that 'I am moving my hand' as opposed to 'This hand is not in my control'.

We have raised several possibilities: (a) Robert thought that the movement of his left hand was not caused by him because the right hemisphere that was responsible for this movement did not have conscious awareness; (b) the right hemisphere did have awareness, but this could not be communicated because such an act requires the medium of language, which was dissociated from and therefore not accessible to the right hemisphere; (c) the right hemisphere does have awareness of certain functions, such as emotion and artistic appreciation, but not language and movement, the awareness of which is a property of the left hemisphere. These are only some of the hypotheses that account for the observations that have been made in split-brain patients. What was strange, however, was that the left hand often moved when Robert was moving his right hand, then performed a conflicting act. At times, there was even an impression that the two hemispheres were in conflict, playing out a Freudian drama that had swelled to the surface rather than being constrained to the deep recesses of the unconscious.

There is a plausible 'scientific' explanation for the intermanual conflict (the left hand interfering with the activity of
the right) based on our understanding of the process of brain
activation when an action is performed. The movement itself
is the direct result of activation of the motor cortex, a strip of
brain tissue forming the posterior border of frontal lobes and
communicating with the opposite limb. Activity in this part of
the brain is necessary for voluntary movement to occur, but
the process does not start here. Even before the motor cortex
is activated, neurones lying in brain regions in front of the
motor strip, called the supplementary motor area (SMA), can
be shown to be firing. In fact, even when we 'decide' to move
one limb, the SMA is stimulated in both hemispheres.[31] It is
as if the brain is prepared to move both limbs, not knowing
which one will get the final go-ahead and which restrained.
The subsequent activity is such that only one motor cortex is
activated even though the other side may show minor activation. When normal individuals are asked to move a limb, some
muscle activity can be detected in the opposite limb. Activation of one side of the cortex is coupled with deactivation of
the preparedness of the other hemisphere to move. It is likely
that a brain with a corpus callosum section has an inability to
suppress the SMA activity on the unwanted side, resulting in a
bilateral activation of limbs. Activity in the right hand is purposive because it is guided initially by a verbal or other command,
then through visual and kinaesthetic (sensations from joints
and muscles) feedback to achieve a goal. The activity in the left
'anarchic' hand is not so regulated, but it mirrors the activity
in the right hand. In other words, the left hand has been 'told'
to move but, with nowhere to go, it mirrors the movement of

the right hand and therefore interferes with its actions. Robert was able to see the hand move but was unable to command it to stop. To stop the anarchic hand, the activity in the right motor cortex had to be suppressed, and the command for this had to travel from the left hemisphere in which the purposive activity was being generated. The path for this command is normally the corpus callosum, which had now been cut in Robert's brain.

A test of the above theory would be if abnormality in the SMA could produce a similar problem in patients with an intact corpus callosum. Dr Gottlieb and his colleagues from Boston presented cases in which the same phenomenon was produced by partial lesions of the SMA in the absence of callosal lesions.[32] These patients also had problems in one brain region communicating with another, but in this case the pathway affected was in one hemisphere rather than in the connection between the two hemispheres.

The 'alien' hand, moving because of the unsuppressed activity in the SMA and therefore the motor cortex, is therefore a victim of a lack of normal suppression of movement on the other side when we move a limb, something that is part of our normal physiology. Is it appropriate to consider it 'interfering' or 'vicious' or 'malevolent'? Does the movement of the left hand indeed have a nefarious purpose? It seems that the attribution of a purpose is after the fact, a 'rationalisation' by the observing and disapproving left hemisphere. The observation that a part of our own body is moving autonomously can be deeply disturbing, and it is quite likely that we will attribute an aggressive or destructive motive even when no such intention is present. There are some patients with the alien hand who deny the presence of a left limb, disowning it altogether and treating it as a foreign body. These patients have brain lesions that extend beyond a simple corpus callosum section to parts of the brain involved in the formation of the concept of self.[33] There is much evidence that the prefrontal cortex, the front part of the brain so important for our highest mental functions, has an important role to play in this. The alien hand syndrome can therefore take different forms depending upon which other brain regions are affected. A surgeon's knife generally delivers a clean cut of the corpus callosum, but even in these cases, other brain regions are often abnormal because the individual suffers from epilepsy. When the corpus callosum disconnection is due to a tumour or lack of blood supply, the abnormality usually extends to the neighbouring brain regions.

This seems to be an appropriate place to introduce two other inter-hemispheric connections, the anterior and posterior commissures. A commissure is in fact a place where two things are joined, and the corpus callosum is one large brain commissure. Both in front and behind the corpus callosum are two smaller fibre tracts that connect the two hemispheres, the anterior and posterior commissures. There are also some connecting fibres in the hippocampal region (hippocampal commissure) and middle of the brain (supraoptic commissures of von Gudden and Meynert) that are less well known. The anterior and posterior commissures are less than a tenth the size of the corpus callosum, but do have important functions, and can compensate for the loss of traffic due to corpus callosum section. Interestingly, a flurry of debate was created in 1991 by the finding by two scientists from the University of California in Los Angeles that the anterior commissure is a third larger in men with homosexual orientation.[34] The argument presented was that homosexual men had brains in which the two hemispheres had better cross-talk and, in this manner, they resembled the brains of women more than men. Needless to say, much controversy exists on this topic.

Robert's hand did not continue to behave in this manner indefinitely. The problem lasted only a few days, and he then demonstrated increasing control over his left hand and the intermanual conflict ceased. Had the brain repaired itself? He still found the left hand clumsy and was unable to perform complex tasks with it, but it no longer had its own will. 'It belongs to me once again,' he said in a lighter vein. This happy outcome is usual in patients with corpus callosum sections, but there are other patients who continue to experience the alienation of their limbs for long periods. What is different about these patients? It would appear that the latter have abnormalities in other brain regions as well, particularly in the frontal lobes. Is it possible that the transient alienation we saw in Robert's case was in some way related to a temporary injury to his frontal lobes that the brain surgery had produced? We cannot exclude a role played by the frontal lobes, but the consistency with which the alien hand occurs after corpus callosum section argues for it to be the major prerequisite.

Robert now no longer felt that his hand was disposed to anarchy. When tested in detail, there were still tasks that the left hand could not do, but these were subtle, and our neuropsychologist had to dig deep into her bag of tests to bring them to the fore. For all practical purposes, Robert felt that his hand was normal and under his control. He could assert his will. In this case, the basis of the reassertion of his will appeared to be his ability to suppress unwanted activity in his left hand. If free will is the determinant of the carrying out of an act, it has its flip side: that of not acting when the intention is not to act. It is very often this inability to not suppress a movement, or not act when not wanting to, that is the more prominent determinant of volitional activity. We can take another clinical example. Patients with Tourette's syndrome have movements like blinking, grimacing and jerking that they can control temporarily but then have to let go. The patient experiences an irresistible urge to move that is not generated by his or her own free will. Such patients acknowledge that the movements are theirs and that they should be able to control them. Their ability to control the movements for only short periods of time suggests to them a 'weakness' of their will. Yet they admit that these movements are unintentional. In the case of the tics of Tourette's syndrome, it is the inability to stop rather than the ability to cause that defines the involuntary — or unvolitional — nature of the movements.

Another twist to the neurobiology of free will comes from the research on brain activity that precedes a willed movement. It has been shown that electrical brain waves change several hundred milliseconds before the conscious decision to move, as if the brain is anticipating the decision to move. This has been called the 'readiness potential' by electrophysiologists. Some philosophers have argued this suggests that what we call 'free will' is an illusion as 'our choices' have been decided beforehand 'by our brains'. It must be conceded that there is much brain activity beneath the surface that precedes and accompanies any conscious act. The alien hand is testimony to the unconscious workings of the brain, and there are a myriad of other processes happening in the brain that do not reach awareness. The unconscious activity also suggests that the brain has certain predispositions that may determine our behaviour. Some authors argue that the alien hand becomes violent in someone who brings an aggressive temperament to the condition. It does not negate free will, however, as the responsibility of the act is still with the self-aware individual who has not been affected by brain injury. But it does show how fragile this concept of free will really is, and how quickly it can succumb to alterations in brain physiology.

It is remarkable that when I met Robert a year later, he was a confident young man who had shed his pessimism and despair. He still had brief 'turns' that reminded him of continuing electrical disturbance in his brain, but no longer was he falling or losing consciousness. He reported subtle problems in his functioning. He found it difficult to put names to faces, and said that he had to associate special facial features like the length of the nose or the shape of the glasses to a name. His left hand was still a little lazy, and at times his gestures were not in keeping with what he was saying. His mother noticed that she was sometimes surprised by his facial expression because it was not in keeping with his statements. For most people, this was no more than a slight oddity.

How was it that, with such a big lesion in his brain, Robert could go about life as if there was little problem? This is because even with the most complete of sections of the corpus callosum, some fibres may be spared, as in the commissures referred to before, or the brain may adapt some other pathway of communication. We also connect our two brain halves by other means: through our eyes, which feed information to both hemispheres, and through our ears, and touch, and other sensations, which are distributed bilaterally (on both sides of the body and brain) and continue to unite our worlds.

It is probably more than a coincidence that we see similar abnormalities in patients with schizophrenia. The dissociation between emotion and thinking was one of the cardinal features of schizophrenia described by Swiss psychiatrist Eugen Bleuler, who believed that this illness was the result of disordered association between different brain regions. The experience in schizophrenia can extend to a belief that alien forces are responsible for thoughts, behaviour or emotions. The patient may believe him- or herself to be a passive recipient of these forces and feel powerless against them. It has been suggested that callosal pathology may be the basis of schizophrenic illness, but the variety of symptoms, the long duration of the disorder, and the lack of evidence of exclusive callosal abnormality suggests that this is only part of the story. Nevertheless, the callosum, while little more than a bundle of fibres in the anatomist's book, stakes its claim as one of the seats of the soul. Since the soul is not much more than electromagnetic activity in neuronal networks, it is not such a strange idea really. Robert believed that his soul was shaken by his surgery but that it found a new core fairly soon. The ability of the brain to repair itself amazed Robert himself. After so many years of clinical practice, I continue to be surprised by the brain's plasticity. And, indeed, there is hope for every fractured human soul.

3

Swearing like a Spanish sailor

*A sober priest without any eccentricity ... no sign of madness or
any immoderate action (who was said to be possessed by the devil)
... when he passed any church, and genuflected in honour of the
Glorious Virgin, the devil made him thrust his tongue far out of
the mouth; and when he was asked whether he could not restrain
himself from doing this, he answered: 'I cannot help myself at all,
for so he used all my limbs and organs, my neck, my tongue, and
my lungs, whenever he pleases, causing me to speak or to cry out;
and I hear the words as if they were spoken by myself, but I am
altogether unable to restrain them; and when I try to engage in
prayer he attacks me more violently, thrusting out my tongue.'*

Sprenger and Kraemer, *Malleus Maleficarum* (1489)

Tourette's syndrome[1] has long been recognised by an extraordinary set of symptoms: the irresistible urge to utter obscene
words, or think of them obsessively, or to make obscene gestures.
In the last two decades, the scientific writings on this disorder
have been at great pains to de-emphasise this aspect of the
disorder, as it is present in less than a quarter of patients. Some
of the patients of Tourette's might even consider me insensitive
to discuss the symptom of 'swearing' or 'coprolalia' at all. We
now recognise Tourette's by the tics[2] – motor (sudden and only

partly controllable jerks) and vocal (sudden utterances) – and a number of behavioural symptoms: compulsions, obsessions, attentional difficulties, learning problems and conduct difficulties. I agree with this shift in emphasis away from the obscene utterances, which are indeed uncommon,[3] and in no way do they distil the essence of the disorder. But when they are encountered in the clinic, they start the thoughtful clinician on a journey into the dark recesses of the mind where biology, sentiment and culture interweave like vaporous threads.

No one is better suited to send us on such a journey than Amelia, a young woman of Spanish descent who has been the most challenging of my Tourette's patients for many years. She was sent to me by her priest who, having endured the disapproving glances of the Virgin Mary for many months, could no longer bear the wrath of his congregation at the presence of this 'blasphemous' woman who would explode with 'bitch' and 'fuck you' just when the profundity of the mass had sent the church into a poignant silence. The priest had spent a whole Sunday morning talking about this mysterious illness originally described by a French neurologist, George Albert Edouard Brutus Gilles de la Tourette, over a century ago.[4] The foreignness of the neurologist's name had only added to the misgivings of the Church's patrons. Some of them were even convinced that Amelia was possessed and in league with Satan. Her priest did pray for her and, fortunately, did not share this opinion.

The first few minutes of my first session with Amelia and her father, who always accompanied her, as I later discovered, proved to be rather ordinary. She was a plump woman, plainly dressed but with a congenial smile on her face that made her likable, the kind of person one would strike up a conversation with on a train. She had an open manner about her, a certain honesty that made her seem almost childlike and vulnerable. Her father treated her as his little girl who had refused to grow up. They had migrated to Australia when Amelia was 15 years old, and she spoke English like a native Australian, acting as her father's interpreter during the interview. Yet this man, who could not directly converse with me, managed to dominate the initial interviews. Amelia did mention her 'kind' and 'devout' mother a few times, but she never accompanied her daughter for the doctor's visits.

Amelia's story was not unusual for a Tourette's sufferer. Her tics had started at the age of five, around the time her younger sister was born.

'We thought it was attention seeking. You do get a lot of attention if you contort your face like a rubber toy,' explained the father.

'So, the first movements were noted in the face?' I interjected to clarify.

'That is what we first noticed. You know, like an expression of pain, momentarily there, and then gone. We had sympathy for her, but she got her share of punishment for such absurd acts. Her friends would imitate her. Strangely enough, she started imitating us, and believe me, she was serious.'

The imitation interested me. Was her imitation different from that of her friends, as her father seemed to imply, and was it expressed with a different gravity and feeling?

'The friends imitated to tease her,' the father explained. He went on to explain in Spanish, duly translated by Amelia, that she imitated like a driven girl. She seemed to have little control over her need to imitate on these occasions. Her parents even considered the possibility that she was the victim of a possessing spirit.

I wanted to explore further symptoms.

'Then she began to twitch her hands suddenly. These were like convulsions ... We still thought it was her nervousness ... She was a nervous child, somewhat shy at school, and always clinging on to me when at home. On the surface, she seemed peaceful. But when these jerks developed, my wife and I thought that she could not possibly be peaceful deep under ... We tried to keep a lid on things as much as we could ...'

Parental concern increased when Amelia was about 10 years old with the remarkable development of 'swearing'. If they had seen lightning previously, now the thunder had followed. The teachers expressed amazement at this, having hitherto been familiar with a somewhat quiet and obedient Amelia. There were frequent altercations at school, usually provoked by the utterance of an obscenity by Amelia. The particularly distressing aspect of her swearing was the nature of the obscene words.

'I would like to tell you, doctor, but I am ashamed. Not even a Spanish sailor goes this far. I could cut her tongue if I did not love her so much.' I could understand the agony experienced by these God-fearing devout Catholic parents at their daughter's behaviour. 'And she didn't seem to do it in anger or frustration. The words just exploded out of her, like convulsions ... rather like the motor twitches she had at other times ... She had also started making a noise, like a little bark, which was most annoying,' her father explained.

With the family convinced that a spell had been cast on her ('she was cursing because of a curse'), she was taken for what turned out to be the first of many exorcisms. A medical consultation took place around the same time, and the family was told that she probably suffered from Tourette's syndrome. Much like the exorcist, the psychiatrists conducted their own ritual cleansing. One of the first treatments offered was insulin, with injections given intramuscularly every morning five to six times a week until she became comatose. The treatment did not 'cleanse' her mind, and not surprisingly, for insulin therapy had been thoroughly discredited about 15 years earlier and has not been used in Australia for more than 40 years. She was later treated with the dopamine-blocking drug haloperidol (Serenace)[5] with some benefit.

Amelia was 30 when she came to see me, and her 15 years in Australia, except for the first five, which had mercifully been symptom-free, were filled with interpersonal crises. A marriage to a rough, aggressive, alcoholic husband had lasted only two years. 'He swore as bad as I did, except that he was no Tourette's.' She had many jobs, each of which would last a few days, until the Department of Social Security declared her unemployable. 'I could keep a lid on my symptoms for two or three days, but then it became unbearable. I wish there was a job in the middle of the night when all other human beings were fast asleep ... Perhaps I could find work with the deaf ...' She had three hospital admissions and many changes in medication, but with only partial relief. She changed house several times because of complaints from neighbours.

It was not solely her obscene utterances that made her a pariah. Not infrequently following a barrage of abuses ('fuck ... bitch ... fuck ... fuck ... fuck you, prick'), she would bend towards me or her father, and make an obscene gesture with her middle finger, grimacing violently at the same time, as if to reinforce the impact of the statement. As soon as the episode settled, she would apologise profusely, as if the possessing spirit had now departed and the real Amelia was back, being responsible for her actions. Sometimes she would speak under her breath, trying to hide the obscenity and barely succeeding. At other times, it was a dramatic performance, like a satanic ritual for a private audience. She owned it all; there was no suggestion of a schizophrenic split of the ego, no dissociation from this evil side of the self – if such it was – and no invocation of an alien power. Sitting alone in the waiting room, the obscenities were mere volcanic eruptions, bouncing the lava off the bare walls but lacking any direction or meaning except for the spending of some inner force. In the presence of another person, they immediately took direction, as if the animal energy was being channelled by some invisible magnetism. In the presence of her father, the 'cog ue, papa (fuck me, papa)' now only elicited a sad shake of the head from an understanding father. But the word papa was substituted in other situations with devastating results. And the Spanish curses became English ones, depending upon which dialogue was being interrupted. The 'chupa pija' and 'chupa concha' when talking to her father became 'suck prick' and 'suck cunt' when talking to me. It is not without reason that this symptom is known technically as coprolalia (from Greek kopros, dung or faeces, and lalia, lips), and the obscene gestures copropraxia. When Tourette's syndrome was still a novelty, it was often referred to as the 'cursing disease' or the 'foul mouth syndrome'.

My encounters with Amelia took place mostly in the safety of my office. I wondered how her father felt escorting his girl through a supermarket on a Saturday morning, or waiting for a reliably late Sydney train on a busy platform! I requested our social worker Dianne to take Amelia shopping one day and give me a full report. Amelia was not consciously holding back her coprolalia, but the first 10 minutes were blissful – not a trace of the symptom. Then the avalanche came. They were in a busy elevator, trying to avoid encroaching on each other's personal space, when out came a string of abuses: 'fuck, bitch, bitch, you bitch, you … u … u bitch', in a flurry. A dark shade of red went past the countenances of fellow passengers, and a young man could barely muffle a giggle. Amelia noticed him, and out came another string, this time with a rude gesture darted towards him. And then, 'Oh, I'm sorry. Please forgive me. Please forgive me.' Fortunately the lift halted, and Dianne quickly shoved Amelia out, choosing to climb stairs. The storm clouds settled down. Then, while they were waiting in the checkout queue, it happened again, and this time they were less fortunate, because some choice abuses came back with vigour, and a big woman came menacingly towards Amelia. Dianne was forced to give a lecture on Tourette's syndrome while waiting at a checkout counter. And, she told me that it was one of the few times she had wished the ground would split and swallow her whole.

The only person I would have liked her to have met on such an excursion was Sigmund Freud,[6] or one of his disciples. Such an encounter would surely be psychoanalytic dreams come true. Lying bare are the psychosexual entrails of this hapless individual, or so it seems on a superficial examination. Is this anything other than an oedipal drama being played out by a doting and protective father, and a daughter yelling at the top of her voice, 'Fuck me, papa'? And the displacement of these incestuous feelings to neutral figures who are just standing by? The utterances of a coprolalic Amelia fit in with the early Freudian position of a little girl developing incestuous feelings towards her father, turning to him with the hope that he will give her a penis to compensate for her lack of one. The father's response in Amelia's case, the psychoanalysts would argue, arrested her development at the oedipal level. This is reflected in her personality, a histrionic bent towards drama, a sexualisation of relationships, chaotic behaviour and a tendency to emotional outbursts. Amelia was, of course, not conscious of these feelings, and would deny them emphatically if confronted with this analysis. She had 'repressed' them, albeit with partial success. And the tics? They were the converted manifestations of the psychic excitation resulting from the threatening libidinal stimulation. The symptoms were distorted expressions of instinctual impulses that were struggling with an ineffectual repressing agency in the mind. Intermixed with the sexual impulses were aggressive ones, for swearing is more an aggressive than an erotic act. Otto Fenichel,[7] a psychoanalyst whose theories on the psychodynamic origins of tics held sway for many years, attributed the aggressive impulses as originating from the ego trying to repress the infantile sexual impulses. Failing to do so resulted in the aggression being projected on to other people. The impulses then became 'independent of the ego', no longer being part of the personality of the individual.

The above 'psycho'-analysis is as speculative as the much less respectable theory of possession, which was historically the primary explanation for Amelia's disorder. The main problem with the psychoanalytic explanation above, as for many psychoanalytic explanations for neuropsychiatric disorders, is the lack of any substantive evidence. Some aspects of Amelia's personality suggest that a Freudian construction may be a house a theorist can live in, if he or she is prepared to put up with walls that bend when the head turns. There was a certain degree of sexuality about Amelia; to men she often displayed a sign of availability, a certain readiness to consummate a brief encounter. She had at one stage been extremely promiscuous, which had stopped when her father intervened.

Amelia also had another socially abhorrent symptom that I have not yet mentioned: a tendency to touch – not to emphasise a bond, or to communicate a feeling, or to express a wish; in fact, her touching had nothing to do with communication between two individuals. It was another eruption from the dark, unfathomable recesses of her mind; an impulsion to make contact, sometimes on one side, at other times symmetrically on both sides of the confronting individual's face or body. Her touching could surpass her swearing in causing offence. I cannot recall even one occasion wherein I was not conscious of the physical distance between the two of us during an interview. Indeed sliding away or bending backwards to make it more difficult for her to touch me was a common feature. This touching sometimes took a perverse turn. With women, the breasts became targets of this ritual contact, and she elicited such an adverse response from one nurse not familiar with her condition that a staff crisis was precipitated in the psychiatry ward to which she was admitted. With men, an impulse to touch the genitals was resisted only with great effort. When touching others was impossible, she touched herself, first on one side of the body, then the opposite one to even it up. All this because of an 'urge', with no sexual feelings awakening in the conscious mind!

But there was also a non-sexual Amelia – an Amelia who sent Christmas cards with religious regularity, who made jams and pickles for her doctors, who worried for her parents when they were ill, and who wondered with amazement at this other 'person' in her who intermittently exploded to the outside world. It took me many months to get to know this Amelia, bereft of the impulsions that coloured her encounters. Which was the real Amelia? I wondered. I had to agree with her father that she was a 'warm, sensitive, loving, kind and helpful person, who'd rather spend the evening home with her family'. The psychoanalytic theory had not reconciled with the alternative explanation: that her relating to the world was a direct reaction to the way the world related to her. And the world related to her with the mistaken assumption that the impulsions were 'her', the coprolalia was her, the rude finger sign was her; the 'touching', 'cursing' and wicked girl was Amelia.

Is it not true that we see ourselves through the mirror of other people? What, then, had little Amelia known about herself from an early age? Did this girl, who was ridiculed and rejected at every step, see herself as a little monster that would only grow bigger with age? She could not dissociate herself from her impulses; they were her own except that they were alien to the ego. There was no choice but to own them, and occasionally behave as if the real person was a single person, a 'bad' whole that other people thought her to be. Her father knew this, and he knew that he had to protect her from the outside world lest she be physically harmed, for that was all he could do. He also had made her feel loved, and he had succeeded in preserving the genuine Amelia, although this person was available to only a few. He did not care about the psychodynamic theories of incest, for he was a practical man, and a man who could feel for the essence of personhood.

Where are we, then, with the Freudian explanation of her behaviour? To me it is entirely speculative, and falls down when it tries to explain the 'real' person that I have come to know. I can, of course, not 'prove' that it is false, for such is the nature of the Freudian genius that clinical observations can always be made to 'fit'. Sir Karl Popper put it thus: 'It was precisely this fact – that they always fitted, that they always confirmed – which in the eyes of their admirers constituted the strongest argument in favour of these theories. It began to dawn on me that this apparent strength was in fact their weakness ... It is easy to obtain confirmations or verifications, for nearly every theory – if we look for confirmation.'[8]

If we measure the psychoanalytic theory by Popper's criterion of falsifiability, the theory does not stack up to scientific scrutiny. The challenge to us, then, is to offer a more viable alternative. The notion of possession by a spirit would be a viable theory in many societies, but our 'scientific' society finds it unpalatable.[9] Like psychoanalysis, it is not easily falsifiable either. Moreover, the two share a certain therapeutic impotence as far as Tourette's Disorder is concerned. We know that psychoanalytic psychotherapy does not work in Tourette's, and we do not even want to know whether exorcism does.

Could there then be a biological explanation for Amelia's eruptions? Is it possible that her brain has been miswired from birth, such that some circuits have become autonomous and their excitement occurs in complete disregard of the state of the rest of the organ? There is now much evidence that suggests a biological basis for Tourette's and that there is indeed a genetic abnormality that passes down the generations, which finds varied expressions in different individuals. It is not hard to imagine that motor tics can be caused by an abnormality in the brain. We know of many brain diseases in which similar movements occur. The husband and wife team of Arthur and Elaine Shapiro, two New York psychiatrists, are credited with the modern revolution in our conceptualisation of Tourette's syndrome. In their 1988 classic monograph on Tourette's,[10] they list at least 22 neurological disorders that resemble it in their manifestations. And why would some drugs with specific brain action work to suppress the tics if they did not result from some abnormality? However, one question disturbs me: how can a brain disorder make an individual utter obscenities? Is there a 'swear centre' in the brain that can be tapped by disease? Is there a swear impulse that 'normal' individuals can keep in check but the unfortunate Tourette's sufferers fall victim to? We are all familiar with the effects of brain disease on language: a stroke patient's inability to speak, or to understand, or a tendency to produce fluent gibberish. Is there any other outcome?

All of us swear, or have sworn at one time or another. We do it when we are frightened, surprised, disappointed, aggressive or under emotional stress. Swearing is a powerful form of communication, a parsimonious speech with a lasting impact, a blunt weapon that can strike an opponent dumb. Behind its aggression lies a display of confidence and familiarity, a suggestion of being a native. When a young lad migrates to a new country with a different language, among the first words he picks up are swear words, and their competent use tells him, and his peers, that he is home. Let us pose as 'obscenity experts' for a moment and examine the nature of swear words we tend to use. Broadly, there are the obscene words that refer to bodily organs or physical acts ('shit', 'arse', 'fuck', 'crap', 'cock', 'prick', 'piss', 'fart', etc.), and other derogatory words ('bitch', 'nigger', 'wog', 'wop', etc.) that are insulting but are not physical in their associations. Lastly, there are words with religious connotations that can be used as profanities ('God', 'Jesus', 'hell', 'damn', 'holy Mary'). In civil company, profanities outnumber the obscenities. On the other hand, it is most unusual for a coprolalic Tourette's sufferer to utter profanities; their vocabulary seems to be restricted to the first two categories of swearing, as has been shown in a number of studies, including the work of the Shapiros. Could this be because the latter are simpler and more primitive in the neurolinguistic sense? What if a computer with an ability to generate words developed the need to swear? Would it prefer obscenities over profanities?

In the 1970s a computer scientist by the name of William Bennett Jr developed a series of programs to test exactly this hypothesis, using the so-called Markov process.[11] The computer is instructed to produce a string of letters in which the next letter generated is taken from a probability table reflecting the relative frequency of occurrence of each letter in ordinary English. Letters such as E, O and T, which have the highest frequency of occurrence in the language, are most likely to occur in any such string. Lower-order processes use the probability of occurrence of individual letters; higher-order probability tables can be constructed showing the probability of sequences of letters. This process can be used to produce two-letter, three-letter and four-letter strings, and so on. The strings generated by this process show a gradual change, from the lower-order ones being nonsensical to the higher-order ones resembling actual words used in the language. Bennett drew attention to the fact that the second-order and third-order texts had an unexpectedly high number of obscene words. The phenomenon repeats itself if phonemes rather than letters are used to computer-generate words, only more so. A further surprise is in the observation that, as in Tourette's, it is the obscene and not the profane words that are generated by this method. In English, some common obscenities produced are 'shit', 'fart', 'arse', 'fuck', 'cunt', 'whore', 'suck', 'pussy' and 'horseshit'. In German, a similar result is produced.

While this is a clever argument to support the notion that coprolalia 'results from a short circuit in brain functioning that produces high-probability strings of phonemes out of proportion to other words',[12] I am not convinced of its veracity for a number of reasons. It assumes that the computer program is simulating brain processes as far as language generation is concerned. There is no evidence that such is the case. A child does not learn language by the random stringing of probabilistic letters or phonemes, but rather by hearing and incorporating whole words. The storage of language must also be in the form of whole words. A person with memory difficulties forgets whole words rather than some strings, which could possibly produce them. The 'tip-of-tongue' phenomenon is another example – suddenly the memory is jolted into producing the forgotten word. When a patient suffers from a stroke that affects the language ability, 'paraphasic' errors may occur, in which one word is substituted by another, and not by a nonsensical string. Even in the so-called jargon aphasics, the stroke patients who speak meaningless jargon, it is the syntax and the meaning that is lost in their speech, not the ability to produce words. The attempts by the computer are clever but not wise, and they cannot be said to simulate normal speech production. The coprolalic, moreover, does not intersperse the obscenities with nonsensical words, unlike our coprolalic computer.

But does culture not influence coprolalia? Is a Japanese middle-class Tourette's sufferer equally likely to swear as, say, a British aristocrat or a Spanish labourer? Is the Tourette's daughter of an Oxford professor as coprolalic as the son of a Newcastle coal-miner? Would Amelia still have been a cursing Amelia if she had been born in Moscow rather than Madrid? Reports have appeared of coprolalia in different societies. A Japanese study reported that coprolalia was present in only 4 per cent of the Tourette's sufferers in that country. If this low prevalence is indeed the real situation, is it a statement on the Japanese society or its language, or perhaps the two together, for language and culture are hard to separate? But since we do not know the actual prevalence of swearing in most societies – a project that is full of potential pitfalls – the question is hard to answer. More powerful evidence comes from the obscenities used by Amelia – long phrases that could certainly not be conceived to be randomly generated, and the contextual switching from Spanish to English and vice versa, which revealed a hidden awareness of the unintended meaning. And the utterances came with such gusto and ferocity that was reminiscent of the possessed. They had a phonetic quality that had a meaning quite apart from what the obscene words conveyed.

A possible explanation is that coprolalia represents a tic,

and a circuit in the brain is excited, but rather than stringing some nonsensical letters or phonemes, this circuit represents the expression of powerful emotion in the absence of a censor that normally would monitor the appropriateness of the situation. The explosiveness of the utterance gives the censor no time to curtail it, or to substitute a profanity for an obscenity. Such substitution is a common experience: are we not relieved when polite company no longer restricts us from using our favourite obscenity, and no longer limits us to minor profane words? Since it is an aggressive impulse, or another strong emotion, that is being let go, it may come out in accompaniment with a copropraxic sign or a tic or a posture, as it did in Amelia's case. Profanities serve the function of uncorking emotion, but only obscenities serve the additional purpose of aggression, of offence as well as defence. Not surprisingly, Tourette's sufferers choose obscenities. And profanities are certainly more complex psychologically, as they are driven by religious mythology. Obscenities, as we know them, are more physical, earthier, more primitive, closer to the animal tumult that goes on in our brains, and it is these the Tourette's patient makes public. Here is a cauldron that is bubbling, but the lid is weak, and the molten contents spurt out. Both the heating of the cauldron and the weakness of the lid could be caused by biological factors, but culture and background determine what goes into the cauldron.

Do we have any evidence that a neurological disease, other than Tourette's, can cause coprolalia? I am reminded of Arthur, another patient of mine whose curses occasionally fill my waiting room. He suffers from an Alzheimer's type dementia, and his memory and inhibitions have gradually slipped. He is a retired labourer, and his wife says, 'I'd never previously allow this kind of language in my house. When he's drinking with his mates, I can understand, but not in my house. Now I have no control, nor does he.' But his curses lack the Tourettic drama with its explosion and lightning suddenness. Arthur's curses are banal; they do not excite a need to explore and understand, they merely elicit a shrug.

The most fascinating neurological coprolalia cases in the literature, much before our generation of neuropsychiatrists, were those for whom Benedek coined the term 'klazomania'.[13] Many years after having suffered encephalitis lethargica, the 'sleeping sickness' that caused the great epidemic of the 1920s, these patients were found to be jerking, writhing, shaking and prone to multiple tics. Their obscenities resembled those of Tourette's, as if the virus had indeed disinhibited the swear centre in the brain. Coprolalia has been described in other nervous system disorders such as the Lesch–Nyhan syndrome, a rare genetic disorder in which the lack of an enzyme leads to a build-up of uric acid in various body organs, especially the joints, kidneys and brain.

You may well draw your breath at this stage, and say that my argument is no more veracious than the psychoanalytical one that I decried a few paragraphs ago. Have I merely substituted limbic brain circuits for oedipal conflicts, pretending to be more scientific? Are the mysteries any less mysterious because of what I have said? Could it mean that we do not really 'know'? The answer is probably yes, sad to say. Both the psychological and biological arguments we can offer are but meagre attempts to grapple with a complexity we are not fully equipped to handle at this stage of our knowledge. The error may be in our 'need' to have one or the other explanation – either biological or psychological – and to treat them as antithetical to each other. The Shapiros reflect this when they write: 'The available evidence supports the concept that Tourette's disorder is a neurological disorder and, similar to narcolepsy and epilepsy, has no other primary or intrinsic psychological associations, although there may be secondary psychological effects'.[14]

While I am not arguing against the neurological status of Tourette's, Amelia is the perfect example of the poverty of any one simple explanation. The threads of the mind weave through the brain, and to conceive something as psychological is not necessarily incompatible with its being neurological as well. It may well be that the origins are in biology but that the psyche elaborates and accentuates the symptoms and gives them the meaning and significance that is unique to the individual. As Oliver Sacks puts it: 'But whether primary or secondary, reason or rationalization, it is these psychic aspects which confer a sort of absurd "significance" on the tics and relate them to the life and psychic economy of the ticquer.'[15] And the arbitrary dichotomy of mind and body breaks down in the face of such passionate evidence. A 'neuropsychiatry' is born which knows that the mind is but the brain, yet has emerged from it and transcended it.

All psychiatrists, deep in their 'hearts', are monists (believing in the unity of brain and mind) if they ever choose to espouse a philosophy. The shade of their monism may vary with the situation or time, but the mind remains a property of the brain. Yet they act like die-hard dualists when they approach the patient's bedside, reinforcing the antithesis between 'organic' and 'functional' disease, as if the brain exists in one person and is irrelevant in the other. Perhaps they are contemplative enough, or are victims of their own humanism and regard the patient's ills solely as defective interactions between individuals. Their raw data become social and psychological, the techniques of physical science become meaningless in the situation, and the brain does not need to feature. Is it their mistake, or merely a limitation? Or are they fearful of the classic neurologist's fate, whose fascination with pathology and what can be unambiguously established often makes his study of illness bereft of the person he is studying?

We would be afraid to put Amelia in the hands of a physician with a purely biological orientation, whose 'scientific' genius would localise her coprolalia to an unstable limbic lobe and a defective frontal lobe, and fail to understand anything that she had to say through her symptoms. Such a physician would furrow a frustrated brow when the chosen drug did not act, and move on to the next interesting case. Nor could we trust her to one of Freud's chosen pupils, for he would still not admit after five years of therapy that his theories are inadequate when he confronts an unchanged coprolalic in his clinic. We need a Charcot, a Jelliffe, or Sir Denis Hill, both neurologist and psychiatrist, Wernicke and Freud rolled into one! Someone who will give more than a naturalistic picture. Someone who, when dissecting the brain, will not miss the soul. For such a doctor will treat the Tourette's but not miss the person, stop the cursing yet pause to get to know the cursed.

Amelia failed to respond to further trials of medication. I tried her on the full range of drugs used for Tourette's: clonidine, haloperidol, pimozide, risperidone, amisulpiride, tetrabenazine and some others. If she did get some benefit from a drug, it was usually at the cost of intolerable side effects in the form of restlessness, fatigue and poor motivation to do anything. In the end, she would choose to go off medication, or use only small doses to give her slight relief without side effects.

Some patients of Tourette's can be helped with behaviour therapy. Teaching them how to relax can have a beneficial effect on tics, and specific techniques can be used to address particular symptoms. Amelia, like many other Tourette patients, did say that her tics were greatly improved when she was relaxed – listening to music in her own home or playing cards with her father. There are other ways behavioural change can be brought about. I remember a patient with coprolalia who has taught himself to muffle his voice when he utters obscenities so that this symptom has little social impact. He can sometimes cut short the obscene word to a single syllable, which helps him slide over the symptom. I sent Amelia to a colleague who is a cognitive behaviour therapist with much experience in helping patients with Tourette's. Unfortunately, Amelia proved to be too impulsive and prone to sudden changes in the level of her commitment – too 'unreliable', in psychotherapeutic jargon – to give behaviour therapy a good chance of success. This treatment lasted only six sessions after which both therapist and patient were too frustrated to continue.

Amelia's coprolalia has fluctuated over the last few years, and her addresses over this period tell this story. Flats in multi-storeyed buildings, which the Department of Housing is prone to allocate to medical invalids, proved too exacting for her neighbours. The department must be tired of my letters in support of her, and it is by now well instructed in the salient features of Tourette's syndrome. After many failed attempts at housing her, she finally ended up in a house with a court-yard large enough to put some distance between her and the neighbours. She has gradually learnt how to make herself less confronting to her neighbours. She chooses not to hang her clothes in the backyard lest the neighbours' children become privy to her utterances. She keeps her windows down to limit the distance her voice travels. The concerned members of the Tourette Syndrome Association of Australia (TSAA) have visited all her neighbours to reassure them that she is harmless and a victim of her affliction.

Public places continue to pose a challenge. The govern-ment has subsidised her taxi fares, which has made commuting less of a challenge. Her father continues to accompany her to the shopping mall, and in his absence, members of the Associa-tion help out. Her life is not free of incidents, however, and periodically a complaint to the police has to be addressed or an irate stranger has to be appeased. She is a frequent presence at the TSAA meetings, and it is amazing to observe how everyone else is able to ignore her intrusive utterances. I have passed on her primary care to her family doctor and no longer see her in my clinic. I still regularly receive Christmas cards from her, and at any TSAA meeting I attend, I am assured of a kiss on either cheek and a few pats on both shoulders, interspersed with a few choice obscenities and profuse heart-felt apologies.

4

The Mozart complex

All men are creative but few are artists.

Paul Goodman (1911–72), *Growing up Absurd* (1961)

I have always believed that being plain average is a boon. Ordinariness has much to commend it. The expectations others have of you do not reach the sky. If you are aware of your ordinariness, your own ambitions are appropriately limited to match your capabilities. You can look forward to the ordinary pleasures of life with contentment. Since you do not threaten order, few others bother to threaten you in turn. Your days morph into weeks and months, and if you are lucky, this may be your road to contentment.

Why is it then not uncommon to see individuals tormented by their ordinariness? If being 'common' is the sure road to purgatory, why do people want the risky highway of excellence or even genius? It may well be a product of our celebrity society! We are so besotted with the media, especially television, the supreme seducer, that we wish we were 'over there'. The constant exposure to beautiful people on television has made us long ever so deeply for a perfect body. Many of us will spare no expense or pain to undergo that 'extreme makeover'. With the body ever so magnificent, can the brain be far behind?

Andrew was one such tortured soul whose need to escape ordinariness had, through a sequence of events, brought him to the Emergency Room after an overdose. As the psychiatrist on call, I was asked to assess him. By the time I saw him, he had recovered from the acute effects of the many different pills he had taken. It had not been a particularly toxic overdose, and he had not needed any active treatment. The potential lethality of the attempt had therefore been low. I found him to be regretful, and apologetic that he had caused trouble to so many. He was keen to talk about himself. One of the first tasks of a psychiatrist in a situation such as this is to arrive at a diagnosis and assess the risk of a repeat attempt. A treatment plan is then formulated.

In the next half hour, it became quite clear to me that Andrew did not suffer from depression or other serious mental disorder. His suicide attempt had occurred after the break-up of a recent relationship, which had shattered his confidence further and sent him into deep despair. One dominant theme emerged from our interaction: Andrew was unhappy and wanted to better his lot. His life, as he described it, was 'ordinary', and he wanted to break out from being 'average'. The break-up had convinced him that an escape was not likely to be easy. He could see no way out.

I saw him again the following day. I had to agree that his life had 'ordinary' written all over it. His parents, his school, his academic record, his sporting prowess, his musical talent – all had the same word stamped on them. His father was a railway worker, which was a job for life with little expectation but of turning up every morning at the designated time and keeping the trains moving safely. His mother kept a good home and had done her share of tuckshop duty and making lamingtons for charity fairs and school fetes. Andrew was average in his grades, made the second-grade rugby team, and sang well enough to join the church choir. His parents were proud of their 'nice' boy.

Andrew had not accepted that he was a 'good' average in most things. One teacher had taken an interest in him and tried to persuade him that he could achieve excellence by hard work. 'All around you', the teacher said, 'are people who are no brighter or more talented and yet have done well in life. Remember, success in life does not relate highly with your intelligence. Pick an area and work hard at it, and one day you will shine through.' Andrew was not convinced. He could not nudge away the feeling that fate had dealt him a mediocre hand. He could not understand how so many people could be content with their boring lives and appear to be happy. Were they born with a 'contentment gene', or had their parents somehow instilled happiness into them? He thought about his parents – they seemed rather happy with their lives without power or fortune or fame. They sought only the small pleasures in life and thanked God for the little gifts bestowed upon them. Andrew knew he was different – his genes must have suffered a bad shuffle, he thought, or his brain was wired differently. He was now doing a university degree and had psychology as one of his subjects.

He tried to challenge his ordinariness by suddenly dumping his girlfriend and dating an attractive woman ten years his senior. The relationship appeared to work initially. It had given him a level of confidence not previously in his grasp. She had the attributes that he admired: good looks, self-confidence, a well-paying job, independence. He showed her off to his friends – he now had a trophy he could display. The romance took over his life, consuming his waking time as well as his sleep. It was only to last a few weeks. The crash came when she phoned him one day, calling it off without warning. Her reason: she had met someone else more exciting. His overdose followed.

As far as the suicide attempt was concerned, he was not certain that he had wanted to kill himself, and was glad that he was alive. Surprisingly, he was not full of pity for himself. He wanted a future, but one with success. 'They say there is a bit of genius in all of us. Where does my genius lie? I do not wish to be Mozart or Einstein, but is there nothing I can be?' He assured me that he would work hard at it, but he needed my help. Could I assist him in his endeavours? I was uncertain what he expected of me, but agreed to see him for a few sessions to explore the possibilities.

Andrew was not depressed in a clinical sort of way. He had not shown days and weeks of sadness, loss of pleasure, negative ideas, or loss of sleep and appetite. His crisis had occurred precipitously, and he seemed to have climbed out of it quickly enough. When I saw him a few days later, he could smile and engage well in conversation. His body moved with vigour and the demons of depression had no play on his face. His was an existential depression – one that eats from within but may leave the surface unscathed. Clinical psychiatry has no term for this – the convenient label given to Andrew was 'adjustment disorder with depressed mood'. The dilemma that faced me was whether I should explore the depths or merely patch up the cracks on the surface. I am not a psychotherapist by training or temperament, although my psychiatric training has equipped me to explore the human condition. I admire those who embark upon the reconstruction of a broken psyche, but for me it is too long and uncertain a journey. It is not that I am given to the uncontrolled expression of predetermined genes, nor do I underestimate the role of the environment in shaping us. But when I see a finished product – a fully grown man with his frailties and quirks – I become pessimistic about the ability of a psychotherapist to mould his impulses, his selective attentiveness, his emotional valence and his biased cognitions.

I concluded from my interviews with Andrew that all he wanted was to be happy – perhaps not a very profound insight. Is happiness not the ultimate goal of humanity, and indeed psychotherapy? Is that not what mankind has searched for since the antiquities? It had been a simple inference from his behaviour – his suicide attempt – that he was unhappy. He did not refute this when I put it to him. He said that the recent rejection had made him very unhappy, but he had been unhappy to a lesser extent for a long time indeed – perhaps as long as he could remember. 'I was born with the unhappiness gene.' I thought I could clearly see the basis of his unhappiness: the discrepancy between his abilities and his expectations. I was unsure about my ability to lead him toward the path of acceptance of this discrepancy – he might then begin to seek happiness from within and stop comparing himself unfavourably with other people. I could impart simple recipes: to find solace in good relationships, to seek pleasure from giving more than from receiving, to find a higher purpose, to meditate and reflect. To love and to work, as Freud put it! To achieve a balance between yin and yang, as Confucius would have recommended!

I was stunned by Andrew's response – he did not want happiness. 'That would be defeatist,' he argued. 'I do not wish to be happy. Imagine if Mozart had been content being a freak entertainer – would we have *Don Giovanni* or *The Marriage of Figaro*? I am pretty sure Mozart was an unhappy man – he would not have done all he did if he was happy. And thank God he did not see a happiness coach or a psychiatrist!' For Andrew, happiness meant being content with one's lot, an acceptance of his insignificance, a lack of striving for change, a literal status quo. Perhaps Andrew was not ordinary after all. There must be an extraordinary fire burning within him. I put this to him. I did not want his happiness to be a stifling sameness – a lack of growth that he so dreaded. Happiness often dwelled in excellence, and a journey towards excellence could be joyous on the way. My emphasis was to be on the journey itself; so long as it was happy, did the destination matter? Andrew was not so easily convinced.

I had come to refer to his condition as the 'Mozart complex'. The lack of a gift did not mean that his life could not be rewarding. He may not leave a thousand-year legacy, but was that the standard to judge oneself by? I put to him the Mozart dilemma. The genius was flawed. He led a turbulent life and died at 35, sick and poor. Here was the dilemma: what would you rather have – genius or equanimity and happiness? Andrew saw no dilemma in this. He did not believe that Mozart's life could have been anything but fulfilling, and he was unwilling to enter the debate on happiness. 'Can you imagine a mind creating such glorious music to be anything but exalted?' he asked me.

I was perhaps unfairly influenced by the movie *Amadeus*,

which is most likely a distortion of the reality. It is a Cain and Abel story rather than Mozart's biography. Salieri, the Cain to Mozart's Abel in the story, recognised Mozart's genius and helped him in various ways – he even taught Mozart's son Franz Xaver. Mozart's sickness probably introduced a certain degree of urgency in his work, which made him seem desperate. I had of course come across accounts of Mozart's profanities. Were the canons on the words *Leck mich im Arsch* ('Lick me in the arse') and *Leck mich im Arsch recht fein schön sauber* ('Lick me in the arse nice and clean') examples of this? Some had even suggested that Mozart suffered from Tourette's syndrome, although my colleague Professor Mary Robertson of University College, London, did not agree. I was merely pointing out the demons in Mozart's head, real or imagined, to help persuade Andrew of the need for equanimity and balance.

Andrew asked me if I could help increase his mental capacity, his talent and indeed his genius. He had heard of 'neurocognitive enhancement'[1] and the NBIC (neurotechnology, biotechnology, information technology and cognitive sciences) convergence.[2] 'Does modern medicine have something that can enhance my brain?' He was after a technological answer, not a philosophical discourse or a Freudian exploration. 'Is there a drug, or a device, or even brain surgery that can help me?'

'You have come to a physician for help. You must appreciate that my role is to treat diseases. I do not think you have a disease that needs treating,' I quipped.

'I want you to help improve the quality of my life,' he replied.

'Do I then become a quality of life consultant, just like a beauty consultant or a relationship counsellor or a sports coach? I am not sure if I am comfortable with this role.'

Andrew was not aware of the ethical dilemma he was posing for me. He saw me as an expert in drugs and brain devices that may be of help to him. For me, it was not a simple question of enhancing his abilities by some means. The very purpose of the medical profession was in question. I understood the objective of medicine as being that of alleviating suffering. It is what I had been taught in medical school. All enquiries into drugs began with the study of disease mechanisms from which emerged a rationale for intervention. Drugs not designed for such purposes were merely drugs of abuse, to be studied for their adverse effects rather than any potential usefulness. But there was a counterpoint!

When I went to medical school in the mid-1970s, the concept of cognitive enhancement was barely around, although the word 'nootropic' (from Greek, *noos* for 'mind' and *tropein* for 'towards') had been introduced by Giurgea in 1972.[3] C. E. Giurgea was at the Belgian drug company UCB and was the principal researcher in the development of the first nootropic drug, piracetam. The idea behind the development was to have drugs that enhanced learning and increased resistance to the degradation of knowledge in otherwise normal brains by enhancing the flow of information and reducing degenerative processes. Piracetam was hailed as a drug like no other.[4] It was reported to enhance brain metabolism by stimulation of oxidative catabolism and increase of ATP-turnover and cyclic AMP (cAMP) levels, the basic energy molecules in the body. It also enhanced phospholipid metabolism and protein biosynthesis. It reportedly increased the hippocampal release of acetylcholine and the turnover of dopamine, both neurotransmitters being crucial for learning and memory. It thereby enhanced arousal and memory and increased the brain's ability to withstand toxins and other injuries. At least, that was the promise. A number of sister compounds followed: aniracetam, pramiracetam, oxiracetam, all sharing the pyrrolidine nucleus and being closely related to the amino acid, pyroglutamic acid. Amazingly, for drugs with such promising effects on the brain, they were reported to have no adverse effects, even when injected in large doses in animals, and when used in human trials.

Unfortunately, the promise of nootropic enhancement of human ability has not been borne out. The trials in humans have been frankly disappointing, and after the publication of more than a thousand papers, these drugs have not made it into the pharmacopeia in most countries. The claims of many internet companies of the diverse benefits of these drugs as 'safe and effective pharmacologic tools to enhance, protect and optimise truly normal, fully human neuropsychological structures and function, well into old age', lack credibility. I was not going to recommend any of the racetam nootropics to Andrew.

Andrew was familiar with stimulant drugs and wanted to know whether these would help him. These drugs act on the noradrenergic and dopaminergic systems in the brain, which are important for the brain's executive function. These systems help the brain attend to a task, shift attention appropriately to another task, respond in a task-specific manner and ignore competing but irrelevant inputs, or suppress more habitual responses if that is needed. Neuropsychologists have labelled these processes as attention, working memory, set shifting and inhibitory control, and they are the processes that are disrupted in attention deficit hyperactivity disorder (ADHD). No wonder stimulant drugs such as amphetamine (Dexedrine, Adderall) and methylphenidate (Ritalin, Concerta) are routinely used to treat ADHD. There is extensive evidence that stimulants help some individuals, both children and adults, who suffer from ADHD. The question uppermost in Andrew's mind was whether the drugs would help him even though he had not been diagnosed to suffer from ADHD.

I am reminded of Steve, a patient in our clinic for ADHD. From his preschool years, he was his mother's nightmare. If there was trouble a young child could get into, Steve was there. If the front door was left unlocked by oversight, the next couple of hours were predictably spent looking for Steve in the neighbourhood. A trip to the Emergency Room at least monthly was assured, for sutures for a gash or a cast for a fracture. It never ceased to amaze the doctors how dangerous Steve's backyard was even though his father had removed every conceivable hazardous object. When Steve's mother became sick, she discovered that her medicines had all been poured into one large concoction. His baby brother had to be protected from being pinched and prodded or fed magic potions. When Steve was finally packed off to preschool, his mother discovered that she now had to spend much of her time at the preschool, trying to appease the teachers and irate parents of other children. Steve was a real-life Dennis the Menace.

Steve's subsequent ride through life had been a very bumpy one, and his hapless family had no choice but to go along. He encountered disciplinary problems at every step. He was the child known to give other boys black eyes, his clothes were frequently torn in fights, he was detention personified at school, his handwriting was the worst in class and he was behind in his academic attainments. He struggled from one 'does not apply himself and can do better' report card to another. He did show some sparks of brilliance. He was quick witted and had an excellent vocabulary, something that got him out of trouble in many places. He was also exceptional at fixing things, arriving at solutions quickly and almost effort-lessly. After scraping through school, he became an apprentice plumber, then self-employed as a plumber. This proved to be tumultuous, his work record becoming a litany of complaints about unfinished jobs, missed appointments, unpaid work and no tax returns. The situation changed only when he married Alison, who realised the seriousness of his disorganised exist-ence and took charge of the planning and documentation of his business. She provided the structure for his work and life that he clearly lacked. All through these years, the diagnosis of ADHD was never discussed. Many years had passed, and in Steve's son, appropriately named Dennis, now aged five, he saw his story repeating itself. Dennis was taken to a paediatri-cian and diagnosed to have ADHD. Steve and Alison wondered whether Steve did not suffer from the same problem and whether he could still he helped. They found out about our clinic for adults with ADHD.

Steve's story had a somewhat happy ending. He was treated with Ritalin, and for the first time he felt that his thought proc-esses had slowed down. He could now sit and think through a difficult situation. He could apply himself to a task to its completion, and found that his desk was tidier, he had fewer arguments with his wife and child, and he was more relaxed. Ritalin had been magical for him. I saw him a year later, and he still felt that to take the drug had been the best decision in his life. Of course, this was not the most common story in the clinic, and many patients improved very little, or only for a short period. In Andrew's case, there was no indication that he suffered from ADHD, and the role of stimulant drugs such as amphetamine and methylphenidate (Ritalin) was quite unknown.

Amphetamine has been around for more than a century, having been first synthesised by Lazar Edeleanu at the University of Berlin in 1887. It is closely related to a naturally occurring substance, ephedrine, and was considered to be entirely synthetic until 1997 when it was isolated from an acacia species native to Texas (*Acacia berlandieri*).[5] It comes in two optical isomeric forms: D- and L-amphetamine, both of which are psychoactive and act by binding to the proteins for the transport of dopamine, norepinephrine (noradrenalin) and serotonin, neurotransmitters involved in cognition and emotion. The result is the increased availability of these chemicals for their action on the neurons. D-amphetamine (Dexedrine) acts preferentially on the dopaminergic system, increasing alertness and reinforcing behaviour, while L-amphetamine is more active on norepinephrine. Amphetamine is known to be transported into the cells, where it facilitates the release of dopamine with the nerve impulse. In 2001 another group of neural receptors, called the trace amine–associated receptors (TAAR),[6] were identified, and amphetamines act on these receptors. The significance of this finding is, however, not known at present. Methylphenidate has pharmacological actions very similar to amphetamine.

Do the amphetamines help people not suffering from

ADHD? The ability of stimulants, which include caffeine, to increase alertness and wakefulness has been exploited by students before examinations and truck drivers on long-haul transportation. That these drugs can keep you awake is not in dispute. Do they make you perform better when you are so 'awakened'? It is surprising that compared to the scores of studies of stimulants in patients with ADHD, only a handful of studies have examined the drugs in healthy individuals. One such study was published in 1997 by a Cambridge (UK) group.[7] They gave 28 healthy young adults methylphenidate 20 mg/40 mg or placebo in a double-blind counterbalanced manner, and tested them on a number of neuropsychological tests about 1.5 to 2 hours later. Methylphenidate improved performance on some tests, in particular those that involved spatial working memory (the ability to keep pictures or images on line in the brain) and planning. Interestingly, this happened only when the drug was given first and therefore the task was novel. If the drug was administered after the placebo, so that the participants had already been exposed to the task once, they were quicker to act, but their performance accuracy went down. In another study by the same group,[8] healthy young people performed better after taking methylphenidate on the Tower of London test. This is a classic test of planning in which two boards are presented, each with a number of pegs and coloured beads. The individual doing the test is required to move the beads on the left board to match the arrangement on the right, in as few moves as is possible. Brain imaging studies have shown that the left frontal lobe is the brain region involved in this task.

These studies attest to the complexity of the effects of the drug on cognitive processes – a simple conclusion that the drug makes you smarter is way off the mark. You must pay particular attention to the nature of the task that must be influenced and whether this must be done once or repeatedly. We do not, in fact, have good information on the effects of the drugs when they are used over a period of time. The students using the drugs on the night before their examination know one thing for certain – the drug will keep them awake so that they can study their books. They have not thought through the question whether the drug will help them retain the information better and to use it creatively in the examination. Even more importantly, they do not know that by the time they reach the examination hall, the drug effect might have waned, and what effect this might have on their performance. Would they be amotivated or feeling low? Is it possible that information acquired during a drugged state may no longer be accessible when the levels have dropped to zero?

I was certain what my response to Andrew should be – I was not willing to prescribe a psychostimulant drug to him to enhance his brain. 'Not only is it illegal to do so in Australia but also I am not convinced that it will help you, and I would be exposing you to a number of health risks.' The Hippocratic dictum was deeply ingrained in me: 'First, do no harm.' I was happy for him to stimulate his brain cells with caffeine, although I warned him that he could overdo this as well.

There is of course the promise of a new class of drugs called the eugeroics (literally, 'good arousal'). The best known of this group is modafinil (Provigil, Alertec or Modavigil), which Andrew had heard of as another 'smart drug'. When investigators at the University of Cambridge administered this drug to a group of healthy individuals, it increased their alertness,

attention and level of energy.[9] Its mechanism of action is different from that of the psychostimulants. While it does increase
the levels of dopamine and norephinephrine at the neuronal
transmission level, it does not produce the euphoriant effect
of stimulants, and its withdrawal is not followed by a crash.
Its effects are more subtle, and its wakefulness has the feel of
being natural. This may be related to its actions on another
class of proteins in the brain, called the orexins or hypocretins.
They are involved in the regulation of the sleep–wake cycle,
and deficiency of orexin is responsible for the disorder called
narcolepsy in which individuals have an irresistible urge to
sleep, literally at the wheel. In fact, treatment of narcolepsy is
the main indication for the use of this drug in most countries.
Modafinil reduces the experience of tiredness and sleepiness
after sleep deprivation. Defence forces are interested in it for
elite troops who have intense operations lasting a few days
during which they can afford to sleep only for short periods. It
will allow a person to be awake for 48 hours or so, then sleep
normally without having to pay back the sleep debt. John A.
Caldwell of the US Air Force showed that dexamphetamine
could reverse the decremental effects on performance of 40
hours of sleep deprivation,[10] and modafinil could achieve the
same. Modafinil has been reported to help the tiredness and
amotivation of depressive disorder. The drug must, however, be
seen for what it is: something promoting arousal in a manner
closer to normal wakefulness, but not a drug to make you
'smarter'. To label it as a smart drug would be an error.

I thought of other drugs that had been used for enhancement. What about Prozac and other serotonergic drugs? Prozac
was one of the drugs that had transformed modern psychia-

try. The compound fluoxetine was developed by researchers with the drug company Eli Lilly to target the neurotransmitter serotonin specifically.[11] There was accumulating evidence to suggest the role of serotonin in mood regulation, and the researchers wanted to develop a drug that was a specific serotonin reuptake inhibitor (SSRI), thereby increasing the level of this neurotransmitter at the receptor. When the drug was first introduced into the USA market in 1987, it created quite a stir and quickly captured the imagination of the mental health profession. However, its claim of being the first SSRI was historically inaccurate. The drug zimelidine had previously been developed by the Nobel Prize-winning Swedish pharmacologist Arvid Carlsson, and the drug Fluvoxamine, another SSRI, had been introduced in Europe in 1983.[12]

Nevertheless, fluoxetine (Prozac) took the USA and later the rest of the world by storm. Psychiatrists were glowing about its safety and how it would transform the care of depression. It began to be promoted for anxiety, panic, phobia, obsessionality, shyness and low self-esteem. Testimonies to its transforming nature were published in the lay press. The popular book *Listening to Prozac* by the psychiatrist Peter Kramer summarised this very well.[13] Prozac was being used to change personality, with claims that it made the person bolder, less sensitive to social rejection and more willing to take on risks. It was promoted by many as a cheap alternative to the couch. Its sales soared in the billions of dollars, and a number of 'copies' were introduced. After such hype, there was of course the inevitable fall. Reports of suicide and homicide, and the inability of some individuals to stop the drug without disabling symptoms, led to a flurry of medical comment, law suits and soul searching.

I had used Prozac and other SSRIs in the clinic for patients who suffered depression, anxiety, obsessive compulsive symptoms, phobias, social inhibition and panic attacks. Andrew did not qualify on any of these grounds. Prozac was by no means a smart pill, and there was no hope that it would light a spark of genius.

What about drugs for cognitive disorders such as Alzheimer's disease? The list of drugs with claims of anti-ageing and anti-degenerative effects is long indeed. I have met many individuals who are religious about their intake of gingko biloba or brahmi or some other herbal preparation. Brahmi, from the plant *Bacopa monnieri*, has been used in the traditional Indian Ayurvedic system of medicine for thousands of years as a brain tonic, but the scientific evidence in its support is weak. Gingko is a Chinese herb that has again been used for its healing properties for many thousand years.[14] While some studies supported its ability to enhance memory in Alzheimer's disease, a large trial by the National Institute of Health in the USA did not find it to be helpful. Others have claimed that their regular intake of B vitamins or lecithin or inositol or fish oil keeps them in good nick, physically and mentally. Some drugs that dilate the blood vessels and increase blood supply to the organs have been promoted for their cerebral enhancing effects. Hydergine, an ergot preparation, was claimed to 'increase intelligence, memory, learning and recall', among other benefits.[15] Scientific evaluation of the drug has resulted in no support for its clinical use. Inositol is said to promote some neurotransmitter pathways involved in signalling in the brain, and was enthusiastically studied for depression and Alzheimer's disease. But its fan base is quite thin. Since calcium channels play an important role in the healthy functioning of neurons, drugs that block these channels (nimodipine, verapamil and nifedipine, for instance) were studied, with encouraging effects on memory in aged rats that did not translate equally well in aged humans. This long story has a short ending: none of these drugs have clinically demonstrable benefits in humans. Many of my patients with early Alzheimer's disease or age-related memory problems continue to take these drugs, in the absence of any clear benefit. They cling on to the hope that perhaps the drugs help a little, and so long as they do not produce serious adverse effects, I choose not to take their hope away from them, considering our relative ignorance about their long-term effects.

Drugs that act on acetylcholine (ACh) have received much attention in recent years. ACh has been touted as the memory molecule, which is only partly justified. In fact, it was the first neurotransmitter to be discovered in the early twentieth century, and has a variety of actions. Of interest to memory researchers is of course the finding that blocking its action in the brain leads to memory impairment. A natural substance that blocks its effect is atropine, derived from the plant 'deadly nightshade' (*Atropa belladonna*). Atropine of course has many effects on the body, testifying to the diverse effects of ACh. Medical students remember poisoning with atropine to result in 'Hot as a Hare, Dry as a Bone, Red as a Beet, Mad as a Hatter, Blind as a Bat'. Atropos (the Inflexible) was one of the Three Fates in Greek mythology, and the one who chose the mechanism of death of each mortal. She cut the 'thread' by which each life hung; the thread had been spun by her sister Clotho (the Spinner) and measured by the other sister, Lachesis (the Apportioner). Incidentally, *belladonna* is Italian for 'pretty girl', and it is said that Cleopatra used atropine to dilate her pupils to make herself look more beautiful. Atropine, when acting on the brain, produces not only amnesia but also visual hallucinations and agitation. A sister alkaloid is scopolamine (hyoscine), a potent drug known for its mind-altering properties due to the blockade of the cholinergic receptor, thereby blocking the action of acetyl choline. It is often mistakenly referred to as a 'truth serum', and it is alleged that the notorious Nazi doctor Josef Mengele experimented with it to interrogate prisoners. It has many references in the literature and films, which include Robert Ludlum's *Matarese Dynasty* and the classic film *The Guns of Navarone*.

Our interest is more in increasing ACh in the brain to see if it would improve memory. There is good experimental evidence that an alkaloid called physostigmine – obtained from the Calabar bean – increases the level of ACh in the brain by blocking its metabolism, and temporarily improves memory in rodents and in human volunteers. This has been the rationale for the introduction of drugs like donepezil, rivastigmine and galantamine for the treatment of Alzheimer's disease, which have found world-wide acceptance. These drugs inhibit the enzyme acetyl cholinesterase, which is responsible for the degradation of ACh, thereby resulting in increased availability of the neurotransmitter. But do these drugs help memory functioning in healthy individuals? In an interesting study, a team of researchers from Stanford University administered donepezil for one month to pilots and tested their performance on Cessna 172 flight simulation tasks.[16] When on the active drug, the pilots performed much better, especially in emergencies, as compared to the placebo. Did it mean that I should prescribe donepezil to healthy individuals to increase attentiveness? The evidence is too scant for this to be a confident recommendation. We do not know whether this experimental benefit translates into a real-life situation and how long the benefit, if any, would last. The drug is not without side effects, and the cost-benefit ratio might still be against its use. The equation is different when it comes to Alzheimer's disease as we know that in this disease, the cholinergic system is defective and in need of assistance if it cannot be repaired.

In the Memory Clinic at Prince of Wales Hospital in Sydney, my colleagues and I have witnessed many successes and failures of cholinesterase inhibitors, as the above drugs are usually known. I can recall George, who came to us with problems with his memory. At 72 years, he was still running his clothing business, but cracks had begun to appear in various places. He had difficulty remembering the names of his customers. He sometimes stared vacantly at his employees, knowing who the person was but being unable to recall the name. He would get hopelessly intertwined when writing a quotation, and would have to turn to his subordinates to sort things out. At home, his family had become familiar with his questions: 'Where did I put my keys?' 'Have you seen my glasses?' 'Sorry, I left the theatre tickets at work' – these were sometimes the starting points of hilarious interludes or angry exchanges. Then, one day, he had such difficulty finding his car in the car park that he was forced to take a taxi home. This prompted a consultation with the Memory Clinic and eventually a diagnosis of early Alzheimer's disease. He agreed to take donepezil, one of the more frequently used cholinesterase inhibitors, and there was a distinct improvement within a few weeks. The lapses had reduced, he went to work with greater confidence, and he seemed brighter and more motivated to engage with the family. His testing showed improvement in his memory functioning. When I saw him a year later, he had begun to slip again, and was back to the level he had started at. The drug had possibly given him about a year without much deterioration, but since the drug did not prevent further decline, its benefit was only temporary.

Memory enhancement should make a person smarter in some tasks even though memory is only one aspect of intellectual functioning and does not have a high correlation with creativity. Individuals with good memory do well academically because academic learning involves remembering. Scientists have tried to understand the memory processes at a molecular level to provide a rational mode of intervention. Two kinds of processes are relevant for this: an initial event that relates to the induction of memory, and processes that involve its consolidation. The induction of memory involves calcium currents in the neurones, which are due to increased activity on glutamate receptors, especially the so-called AMPA-type receptors. Drugs that modulate the activity of these receptors are called ampakines, and the race is on to find the best drugs for this function with international pharmaceutical companies such as Cortex, Organon, Servier and Eli Lilly being involved. There are a number of promising candidates, but of course we have to wait a few years before any of these become clinically available.

It has been known for a long time that the conversion of short-term memory to long-term memory involves the formation of proteins. The work of Eric Kandel and Paul Greengard at Howard Hughes Medical Research Institute in New York showed that one of the proteins involved in this process was the cyclic AMP response element binding (CREB) protein, which helped neurones form new connections or synapses. Fruit flies with a gene modified to increase CREB protein show amazing spatial memory. CREB may also be important for the survival of neurones. Not surprisingly, scientists began work on drugs that might modulate the activity of CREB16,[17] and at least two biotechnology companies (Helicon, Memory Pharmaceuticals) are pursuing this strategy. Memory Pharmaceuticals was in fact founded by Nobel laureates Kandel and Gilbert, and has a compound labelled MEM 1414,[18] among others, that has shown potential. These drugs have the fascinating promise of being true memory pills, even for healthy individuals, but whether they will come with adverse effects is not known. For example, CREB activity is ubiquitous in the body, but for memory, only the temporal and frontal lobes of the brain are of interest. Will such target selectivity be possible with the drugs, or will there be unacceptable side effects? Only time will tell.

At this stage, these drugs offer tantalising promises, but there was nothing I could prescribe that I was convinced had been tested and found to be effective. I explained to Andrew that as far as cognitive enhancement was concerned, he had come to me a few years too early.

Can direct brain stimulation be used to enhance its performance? The mention of brain stimulation fills most people with awe as well as dread. If there are ways of directly stimulating the brain, they must surely carry the potential of influencing

thoughts and emotions. The dread stems from images of electroconvulsive or shock therapy (ECT) with all its negative
publicity through the media. Transcranial magnetic stimulation
(TMS) is one technique that has recently attracted much interest. TMS directly stimulates the brain using a powerful magnetic
field but without inducing a seizure, unlike ECT wherein it is
necessary to induce a generalised seizure. TMS was introduced
into psychiatry as a potential non-convulsive brain stimulation
technique, and has shown early promise. Neuropsychologists
have used this technique to study brain function and, interestingly, a few reports suggested that it could temporarily improve
brain function. Stimulation over the frontal lobes can improve
the time taken to respond to some tasks. My colleague, Professor Alan Snyder from the Centre for the Mind at the University of Sydney, went even further and suggested that using
TMS to block a brain region might paradoxically increase a
person's creativity. The theory behind this is that creativity seen
in childhood is normally inhibited as the brain matures and
becomes more 'rational', and this may be related to activity in
the temporal lobe. Magnetic pulses administered repetitively
to this brain region will result in temporary reduction in the
activity of this brain region, thereby releasing the buried creativity in the brain. He conducted a study to prove this, but the
results were not completely convincing.

The idea of shutting off a brain region to release creativity, while paradoxical, is not without scientific basis. Professor
Bruce Miller, a neurologist at the University of California at
San Francisco, has described a number of patients with a special
kind of dementia called fronto-temporal dementia (FTD)
who showed evidence of creativity for the first time when

their brains began to suffer from degeneration. One patient,[19] a successful businessman, began painting for the first time at the age of 56, having shown no interest in art previously. The initial paintings were rather simple, featuring brightly coloured shapes. Over the next few years, the drawings became clearer and the colours harder, and he would spend long periods of time getting them right. The quality of the pictures was good enough to win him awards at local art shows between the ages of 63 and 66 years, although by 67 his work began to deteriorate. His dementia had progressed alongside his artistic pursuits. In retrospect, he was showing early signs at the age of 56. At 58 years, he had clear evidence of dementia with problems in language and disinhibited behaviour. (He was noted to change clothes in parking lots.) A feature of his dementia was a heightened awareness of colours and sounds in the environment, on which he frequently commented. By the age of 68, he had deteriorated so much that his artistic talents could not override the loss of expressive abilities of his brain, and he drew bizarre doll-like figures only. Investigations of his brain showed deterioration in the front part of the temporal lobe on both sides, with the right side affected more than the left. The authors speculated that deterioration of this part of the brain resulted in heightened visual awareness in this man, which provided strong motivation for painting.

Another patient described by the same group of investigators was a high school art teacher with training in traditional Chinese brush painting as well as Western watercolour, which she had combined to good effect.[20] In 1985 she showed the first evidence of cognitive problems when she started having problems in planning her lessons and grading the class, and began to rely on her son. Between 1990 and 1993 her artistic productions changed, and she produced exquisite highly patterned paintings based on Chinese horoscope icons. In 1995 she could no longer continue with her teaching and resigned. However, she continued to paint, and in 1997 and 1998 produced some of her best work. While this was happening, her language was deteriorating and her social skills were being compromised. When she was assessed in 2000, she had stopped driving and writing, and her language output was minimal. Her frontal lobe functioning was also compromised. She was diagnosed to have an uncommon form of fronto-temporal dementia known as progressive aphasia, in which language function deteriorates progressively due to frontal lobe atrophy until the late stages when other cognitive functions become affected as well. The authors argued that her dementing disorder had freed her from the constraints of her formal training as well as societal expectations, and this had resulted in the emergence of free expression of an emotional style. This belief is held by many – society, through its process of socialisation, curbs our inherent artistic talent and freedom of expression. To put it simply, our society has become dominated by functions of the brain's left hemisphere, with its rationality and planning. This patient was, later in her life, freed from this by degeneration predominantly of her left frontal lobe. Similar cases have been described by others. The abstract expressionist painter Willem de Kooning (1904–97) showed a change in his style later in life, becoming freer and simpler in his paintings. He was greatly productive in the 1980s, which was the time he started showing signs of memory impairment, and was diagnosed with Alzheimer's disease in 1989. His later paintings, however, lost their uniqueness and were more like each other.

If brain disease can sometimes unleash creativity or enhance it, can an argument be presented to create brain lesions to promote artistic expression? Many individuals would recoil at the very idea. We must accept that disorders such as dementia are quite common, but artistic expression under their influence is a rarity. It must therefore be the consequence of a particular set of circumstances coming together – possibly a predisposition combined with a compulsive urge that is allowed to express itself while the brain has many capacities preserved. How an artificially created lesion can replicate this state in an individual is impossible to answer at this stage. No one would be reckless enough to create a surgical lesion in the brain of a healthy person with the expectation that it would unleash creativity. A medically acceptable technique, however, is TMS because the magnetic pulses can temporarily create what can be called a 'virtual lesion' – transient dysfunction of a targeted brain region, which produces no lasting effects. The experiment by Alan Snyder[21] showed a hint of this being successful in a few individuals, although the technique is still too crude in relation to the complexity of brain circuits for this to be a reliable method.

It will be clear from my musings that I would not make a very good lifestyle consultant. It is true that lifestyle gurus are not prone to the kind of doubts that scientific training is designed to inculcate. They do not groom the evidence with the same fine teeth. Thankfully, the promise of vast riches from such consultations will not take the physician–scientist out of me or my like-minded colleagues. I had laid bare to Andrew the limitations of science. I had also become aware of some conflicts that had continued to trouble him. I offered him the possibility of psychotherapy with a colleague who was skilled at dealing with such problems. He was uncertain about it but agreed to consider it.

I had thought I would never see Andrew again. I was surprised when three years later, he made an appointment to see me again. He had not come with a medical problem. The only purpose of his visit was to tell me that he was happy. He had brought his charming girlfriend with him. He had a job with a marketing company and had gone back to university part time. He was grateful to me for our brief encounter some years ago and had come specially to thank me. He told me that he had mulled over our discussions for many weeks, then taken up the referral to a psychotherapist whom he saw for about a year. His life's travails had gradually become clearer to him. He had gone on to read a number of books on success and happiness. He believed that although on the surface he was not very different, his life had transformed in this period.

I wanted to find out what he thought the secret of his transformation was. Was it because he had found a good partner? Was it that he had discovered his inner strength? Had he accepted his position in life? His answer was quite unexpected. 'I have learnt that the secret to happiness is in putting one hundred per cent of yourself into anything you do, be it work or relationships. I do that and my life is fulfilled. I think that was Mozart's genius – he gave music everything he had. For me it is not music or art, but then I was not meant to be Mozart.'

5

The mirror always lies

You can never be too rich or too thin.

Duchess of Windsor (1896–1986)

There is an old saying that beauty lies in the eye of the beholder. No child is ugly in the eyes of its mother. But how is one to decide whether someone is beautiful? Abraham Lincoln is quoted as having said that God must love common-looking people since he makes so many of them. Is it the uncommonness of a face or a body that makes it attractive? The rich and famous are also considered attractive – is it because of their fame and fortune? Research on marriage partners shows that we are attracted to people who resemble us – is it similarity that feeds attraction? Does a child need to be taught who is attractive, or does it imbibe it from the multiple influences its development is imbued in? Could it be that a certain region of the brain signals the attractiveness of a person? The 'eye' may be situated in these neurons, and the 'mother neurons' may be bombarding them with messages of positive bias. Answers to these questions are ambiguous and often couched in metaphor. Poets and artists are not averse to supporting this tyranny of ignorance for the fear that a scientific understanding would peel away the mystery that makes beauty and appearance appealing. Neuroscientists are wary of tackling this problem lest their investigations seem simplistic and on the fringe of quackery.

If beauty has had one object to venerate, it is the human form. Painters and sculptors have known this for centuries. Michelangelo sealed it in his statue of David[1] and Sandro Botticelli in his *Birth of Venus*. Modern cinema celebrated it in Marilyn Monroe and Sylvester Stallone. The human form is the most pervasive of our perceptions – it surrounds us wherever we go. It can also be the private indulgence of a teenager frozen in front of the bathroom mirror. Our conceptualisation of what is attractive, and therefore worth attaining, has differed through history, but modern society has become fixated on the lean frame, especially for women. In Western societies, feminine beauty has become synonymous with thinness. It therefore seems unsurprising that the desire to lose weight and be thin becomes manifest in the preadolescence years and reaches a pathological crescendo in a few unlucky young women.

One person caught in the thinness trap was Annabelle (known as Anna[2] to her friends) whom I first met when she was 19 years old and in her first year of an arts degree at the university. Not having great expertise in treating anorexia nervosa myself, I was not generally referred such patients – she was in fact being seen by my colleague who ran an eating disorders service in another hospital. He was intrigued by an observation that many clinicians have made in the past: the body image disturbance of anorexics. Anorexic women see themselves as fat and cannot bear to look at themselves in the mirror or to see photographs revealing their contours.

This was true about Anna as well: she said she was fat. One

encounter with her was enough to convince me how bizarre this belief was. She had a tall, lean frame. Her face had a chiselled appearance, with prominent cheek bones and large brown eyes. It was heavily painted so that the natural colour of her skin was hardly visible. Her top was loose, giving only a hint of breasts. The jeans were tight, giving her long legs the appearance of two tapering poles. Her face was attractive except for the hollowed cheeks, which might prompt comments like, 'You need to put on some weight.' The extent of her problem became apparent only gradually. When she pulled up her sleeves, the thinness of her arms came as a shock – it was as if the bones could barely be contained by the skin. The skin was covered by a layer of 'baby' hair – usually referred to as lanugo hair and a sign of starvation.[3] She confirmed that she had stopped having her periods about a year ago, and that she had lost a lot of weight over the last two years. 'But most girls would feel OK about that,' she added. 'My parents and you doctors are unnecessarily worried.' She clocked 40 kg on my office scales, and with her 1.65 m height, her BMI (body mass index) came in at 15.[4] A physical examination revealed a very thin body, cold hands and feet, downy hair on her forearms and legs, a heart rate of 55/min and low blood pressure.

Anna had long since crossed the limit of 'fashionable' into the realm of the dangerous. No question, she had severe anorexia nervosa. Her body was in starvation mode. It was clear that hormonal changes had occurred. The sex hormone levels are particularly sensitive to undernutrition, and the ovaries in affected women are quite small. The levels of the stress hormone cortisol are high, suggesting that the body is under significant stress. The immune system is compromised, affecting the individual's ability to fight infection, which can become overwhelming. Anna needed urgent treatment, and I wanted to persuade her to take this seriously.

Her body, when not fully clothed, looked so obviously cachexic that it evoked images of drought ravaged sub-Saharan Africa. It was obviously disconcerting to see her dismissive of the concerns that had been expressed by those around her. 'Can she not see herself in the mirror and be shocked?' I asked myself. In fact I put this to her, and her answer was, for a case like this, somewhat predictable: 'I think I am still a little fat about the hips and the breasts.' 'Which hips and breasts is she referring to?' I thought to myself. I asked her to draw a picture of herself. She drew a quick pencil sketch of a lean girl, with rather full hips and large breasts.

'Is this how you see yourself in the mirror?' I asked, sounding quite puzzled.

'Yes, indeed. But then, I rarely look into the mirror. You see, mirrors can fool you.'

This was an extraordinary aspect of her problem: she could not see the reality about her body form that all else could easily see. The mirror was lying to her. I could not persuade her that her image of herself was quite distorted. When talking about other matters, she appeared quite rational – perhaps a little inflexible for someone so young. She was clearly not psychotic, but her conviction about her body shape bordered on the delusional.[5] This characteristic happens to be common in anorexic patients. Several techniques have in fact been developed to assess the body image disturbance in anorexia.[6] The simplest one, which is the one I used, is to ask the patient to draw a silhouette of their body on a sheet of paper. Instead of this, investigators sometimes hand the patient movable callipers to indicate the widths of various body parts. The same estimation can be done using two light points projected on a screen. Using a special apparatus, one can assemble the estimated parts to form a large silhouette. Of course, with modern technology, one can use various distortion techniques by taking a body form on a computer screen and asking the patient to change it vertically and horizontally until it best matches her conception of her own body. Video distortion methods have been most popular, and life-size projections can be used to make them realistic.

The attention to body image disturbance in anorexia was first drawn by Hilde Bruch,[7] a professor of psychiatry at Baylor College of Medicine in Texas. Various investigators have been keen to find out how deep this disturbance is in the minds of the patients. The first obvious question is: is it present in all patients? The answer is most definitely negative. It is perhaps present in a quarter of the patients – but these may be the most severely affected. The presence of the disturbance certainly is a bad prognostic sign – these young women are likely to have a prolonged illness. Is this disturbance temporary? A fair question, since it is possible that as the patient gains weight, the distortion improves. We recognise that the mental state of the individual can influence their perception of the world and of themselves. An angry person perceives the world as threatening and dangerous; a depressed person undervalues his own skills and attributes. Perhaps the anorexic girl is in a state, owing to her illness, of an altered evaluation of the most meaningful part of herself because she is anorexic and under great pressure from those around her to be different. There is in fact some evidence that as these girls gain weight, their altered perceptions of their bodies do change toward the norm, but the disturbance does not go away in many cases – and these appear to be the ones who are more likely to relapse to their low-weight status.

Do these women actually have a physiological disturbance in their sensory perception? Are they processing the sensory stimuli in the same manner as those with a completely normal eating behaviour and body image? The answer to the second question is most certainly yes. These patients do not show disturbances in other perceptual tasks. They recognise objects normally, can pick ambiguous figures like others, and the physiological examination of their visual systems, using an electrophysiological technique called visual evoked potentials, is normal. Peculiarly, their estimation of body forms of other women is quite normal, even though their judgments are critical. This restriction of the disturbance to their own body form suggests that there must be some difference in the way the body image is being processed in the higher recesses of the brain. The anorexic brain somehow enhances the unattractiveness of the body form, or perhaps focuses unduly on the unattractive features. There is of course a counter-point to this. In 2006 a group of investigators from the Netherlands suggested that the anorexic's body image may in fact be closer to reality, and it might be their healthy sisters who might be overly positive about their own bodies. That is, the bias is in the other group – a positive bias to see your body as more attractive. This, however, relates more to 'attractiveness', that elusive quality that bears only a modest relationship with body form. One cannot get away from the fact that anorexics distort their body form, and see their completely starved bodies as fat.

Being a neuropsychiatrist, my bias is toward examining the brain for an explanation of this disturbance. There is a simple premise underlying this, but one that has endured heated debate over centuries: mental phenomena have their basis in neural phenomena. Even if Anna was processing sensory data quite normally, there must be some difference in the manner in which her brain processed the information about body form when it had been informed that this form belonged to her. This prior knowledge that the form belonged to oneself appeared to be important – the same form, if it knowingly belonged to another, was not distorted in its perception. Anorexic women are critical of fat people and are disparaging of anything that relates to obesity. Their lives are consumed by the desire for thinness, and their food seeking, dieting and exercising behaviour is designed to achieve a low weight. But when it comes to perceiving body form, it is her own body that the patient is likely to distort.

The brains of anorexics have been studied in a number of ways. There have been some interesting reports of brain tumours that were linked to the development of anorexia. These tumours are generally found to affect the functioning of the hypothalamus. This little gland, about the size of an almond, sits below the thalamus – a central relay station – in the brain. The hypothalamus is the central regulator of some of the most important bodily functions such as body temperature, hunger, thirst and circadian biorhythms. For a small brain region, it has a very complex architecture. Two regions of the hypothalamus can justifiably be called the hunger centre and the satiety centre, and abnormalities in these centres can alter eating behaviour. When food normally enters our stomach, some hormones are produced in the gut that signal satiety in the hypothalamus. There are other ways in which the nerve cells of the hypothalamus monitor the metabolic status of the individual. One would, however, predict that if anorexia is being caused by a tumour in the hypothalamus, it will not have the typical cognitive features of anorexia nervosa: the compulsive preoccupation with food, the lying and hiding of food, the purging and vomiting, the morbid fear of obesity, and in particular the distorted body image. This is indeed the case – children in whom a brain tumour was found to be the cause did not have these other features.

Brain tumours as causes of anorexia are of course extremely rare. They are neuropsychiatric curiosities, and while such cases get much mention in the scientific press, they might not necessarily provide us with insights into the more common disorder. Is the brain otherwise normal in anorexia? A finding that has been consistently reported is that the brain of a patient is 'shrunken' – the brain tissue, both grey and white matter, is reduced, and the spaces filled with cerebrospinal fluid are increased in size. This is most likely a consequence of the starvation, with hormonal factors playing a role. As patients gain weight, their brain size also increases, although it might not become 'normal' in all cases. This is of course in comparison with healthy young women, for we do not obtain brain scans on young women before they become anorexic! It is interesting that some women continue to have slightly shrunken brains even after they have gained normal weight, and this could be a sign that complete biological recovery has not occurred.

The structure of the brain, as examined by MRI scans, therefore does not tell us much about the development of the disorder, largely because the scans come in after the fact. Scientists have therefore resorted to the study of brain function. The findings are interesting but not conclusive. Brain cells use glucose exclusively as their fuel for energy requirements, and the examination of the rate of uptake of glucose is a measure of their activity level. Preliminary work shows that the metabolic rates of anorexic brains are comparable to those without anorexia, although there is an intriguing possibility that some regions may be different. Some attention has been paid to two brain regions – the basal ganglia and the hippocampus-amygdala, clumps of nerve cells in the brain that are important for emotion, movement and memory – in which there may be disturbance, but the evidence for this is weak, and it is by no means clear that this disturbance predates the development of the disorder.

A technique that can image the living brain in full flight, while it is engaged in doing a task, is called functional magnetic resonance imaging (fMRI). The principle is fairly simple: any mental task preferentially engages certain brain regions in which metabolic activity is increased as the neurones and their support cells work harder to process the information. This leads to an increase in the blood supply to that region, which in fact outstrips the need for more oxygen in the active region.[8] The oxygen differential between arterial and venous blood in the brain region changes, and this leads to an alteration in its magnetic properties that can be imaged by the MRI scanner. As an example, flashing light repeatedly before the eyes while in the scanner shows an activation of the visual cortex, the brain region involved in perceiving visual information.

Some investigators of anorexia have asked: how does the

anorexic brain process information about food? Zoe Ellison and colleagues at the Institute of Psychiatry in London first published such a study.[9] When six anorexic women were shown pictures of high-calorie drinks (e.g. chocolate milkshake) in contrast with low-calorie drinks (e.g. still mineral water), they experienced an increased activation of certain brain regions, in particular the amygdala, hippocampus, insula and the anterior cingulate on the left side. These findings were interpreted to mean that the anorexia patient's brain is particularly sensitised to stimuli relating to high-calorie food. The amygdala-hippocampus region is involved in signalling fear to the brain, and lays down memories that are charged with negative emotion. The insula is involved in autonomic arousal, and the anterior cingulate in processes that maintain attention. The anorexic patient's brain is focusing its attention on the high-calorie food and producing a fear response akin to the brain of a phobic individual exposed to her feared object. No wonder such foods are diligently avoided by the patient. But the experiment does not tell us when this response developed: did it precede the development of the anorexia or follow it? One can speculate that it probably came first and was the cause of the avoidance of 'fatty foods'. This does not mean, however, that it is innate and a consequence of an abnormal development of the brain. We are beginning to understand how brains develop and what may be the genetic and environmental determinants of deviance in their development. The fMRI study does not necessarily indicate such abnormality and could be a result of deviant learning after the brain had fully developed. It also does not imply that the abnormality is not treatable as, like other phobias, fear of high-calorie food is reversible.

Fear signalling in the brain has survival implications. In the jungle, the fight or flight response determined whether the animal fell prey to a predator or survived to see another day. These emotionally charged encounters were then engraved on the brain, possibly for future reference. But of course, if the response to such negative events persists, it can be quite dysfunctional, as in post-traumatic stress disorder, originally described in war veterans as 'war neurosis'. The slightest noise could make these men jump with fear, and they were tortured by the images of their brutal experiences. The anorexic brain appears to be in a similar mode in relation to food. While it may initially have pay-offs in the form of sexual attractiveness, it quickly becomes the golden cage that Bruch described. Is there a quirk in the anorexia-prone brain that writes in indelible ink? This is quite possible, although we do not know what. It is interesting that Dr Dominique de Quervain and colleagues from the University of Zurich recently demonstrated that the alpha 2b-adrenoceptor, a receptor stimulated by adrenaline – the 'rush' hormone – acts as a gatekeeper of emotionally charged memories in the amygdala, and individuals with one of two variants of this receptor have better emotional memories. A similar mechanism could arguably make some brains vulnerable to the sensitisation of high-calorie food. A partial answer may yet be found in the molecules of the brain.

The trajectory of brain development should also be explored in anorexia. The only way in which we will ever know what brain abnormalities precede the development of the disorder would be if the brains of a sufficient number of girls could be examined before a few of them develop the disorder. This is possible with many of the studies currently in progress.[10] And what about sex differences? An aspect of anorexia nervosa so obvious that it is almost overlooked is that it occurs mostly in young women. Men are not immune to the disorder, but are rarely affected. When they do become affected, the disorder is very similar, with a fear of gaining weight, disturbance in eating behaviour and considering themselves overweight. Why men are resistant to developing this disorder is a mystery. It is commonly believed that this may be because young women are preoccupied with their weight for sociocultural as well reproductive reasons, whereas men do not have such pressures. Young men are more concerned with their musculature, which signifies strength and masculinity in our society. Men who develop anorexia are more likely to have problems with sexuality, which may form the basis of their disturbed body image. One can also speculate that it may be related to sex differences in brain development. The male brain is about 10 per cent bigger than the female brain, and most brain structures display this difference, with a few exceptions. The basal ganglia, especially the caudate nucleus, and the hippocampus are disproportionately larger in women, whereas the amygdala is disproportionately smaller. Having noted the role of the amygdala in fear, might this explain the sex difference in the rates of anorexia? Depression and anxiety are more common in women – could this also be because of brain differences? The basal ganglia have a role in disorders such as attention deficit disorder and Tourette's syndrome, both of which are commoner in boys. The basis for the differences is not known, but may be related to hormonal differences in the sexes. In primates, it has been shown that the amygdala has more receptors for androgens (male hormones) whereas the hippocampus predominantly has receptors for the female hormone oestrogen.

What about the disturbance of body image? Could this also have a basis in brain abnormality? I invited Anna to be part of an fMRI experiment to image the brain while she was examining the body forms of herself and other young women. Ten young women with anorexia with a mean age of about 19 years and a very low mean BMI of 16.4 participated, and they were compared with ten young women with a healthy weight and no history of an eating disorder. While in the scanner, they were asked to focus on two contrasting stimuli, which were digital images of the subject (self) and those of another individual (non-self) matched for age, sex and BMI. All subjects were dressed in standardised clothing (white cropped singlet with abdomen showing, black bike pants and no jewellery), thereby revealing the body contour. All images had the faces pixelated to avoid distraction from body form, with subjects being informed whether it was self or non-self. To make sure that the attention of the subjects was maintained during the viewing of the whole block of 30 seconds, the same body image was shown in three different profiles of equal duration; i.e. front, back and side, changing every 5 seconds.

The results of this experiment were quite interesting. When healthy women were examining images of others or self, their brain activation was very similar. In the case of anorexic women, the activation while viewing other women was similar to that of healthy women. Their brain activation when they were viewing self-images was, however, quite different, with evidence that they were not engaging the brain systems that are usually involved in body image processing, even though they reported looking at the images and were able to rate their responses to the images. In particular, healthy women had greater activation of the insula. The insula is a part of the brain that lies deep on the side at the junction of the temporal lobe and the lower part of the parietal lobe. It is so positioned in the brain that it receives information from multiple sensory modalities: vision, hearing, touch and smell. It has been recognised as a key region involved in the representation of the body schema,[11] and may be crudely referred to as the 'body image centre' in the brain. It is linked with the brain regions that process sensations as well as emotions, and is involved with relating information to the self. Activation of the insula during attribution of an image to self is therefore understandable. The anorexia patients did not show increased activation of the insula. This difference in insula activity between the groups may be a possible reason why patients distort their self-image.

Another region that showed a difference was the medial prefrontal cortex (MPFC), the part of the frontal lobe that sits close to the midline of the brain, and is intimately connected to the regions involved in attention and emotion. The MPFC has been shown to be involved in tasks involving the self; both memory and judgments that have self-relevance result in activation of the MPFC. When healthy women looked at other women there was a reduced signal in the medial prefrontal gyrus whereas there was increased activation in this region in patients. Activation of the MPFC may be related to the metacognitive process of thinking about oneself. The results suggested that the MPFC is being engaged by anorexia patients because they compare themselves intensely with other women's bodies, which reflects the clinical experience.

These differences between anorexic and healthy women might explain why anorexics are so absorbed in their own bodies yet have a distorted view. It raises the interesting question: how do we form an image of our body in our mind? I can close my eyes and see myself in my mind's eye. If someone touches me on a particular part of the body, I know precisely where that happened. I can judge – generally with accuracy – whether a piece of clothing would fit me. I experienced this recently when I was bargain-hunting for clothes in China. The sizes printed on the back of the collar did not match anything I was familiar with, yet I picked the right-sized shirts. When a family friend tricked me by distorting the shape of my body ever so slightly in a photograph, I was quite uncomfortable with what I saw. This must certainly be related to the myriad of exposures I have had to my own body such that I know it like the back of my hand. But surely there is a region in the brain that has this representation as well.

The study of neurological patients proves this beyond a doubt. Julian's story in chapter 9 of this book is one such example: the existence of the phantom limb reminds us of the persistence of the body image even in the absence of continuing sensory feedback from the organ. Quite the opposite can happen in some stroke patients. Peter was one such patient I saw on the stroke ward of the Prince of Wales Hospital in Sydney. He was a 72-year-old bald man with a pleasant smile who had fallen one morning on his way to the bathroom and was unable to get up. When examined in the Emergency Department, he had a clear-cut weakness on the left side of his body: he could not move his left arm or leg at all. When I saw him on the ward two days later, he greeted me cheerfully. In response to my enquiry about his problem, his response still stands out in my memory. 'Doctor, I don't know why I am here. They say I had a stroke, but I am quite all right.' This was indeed odd, as his left arm and leg lay motionless on the side. I asked him if there was anything wrong with his left arm.

'It seems quite all right to me,' he responded.

'Can you please move it for me to see?' I requested.

'Here!' He picked up his left arm with the right hand, then let it fall again.

'Can you try to move it without using your other hand?' I queried.

'Of course I can.' When no movement ensued, he said, 'I am a little tired today. Perhaps you should come back later, doctor.'

The presentation was so dramatic that some of the nurses on the ward thought that he was putting it on. The left side showed all the signs of paralysis. The arm fell with a thud when lifted, and the reflexes were brisk, suggesting a brain lesion. Peter was aware of his surroundings, and his intelligence did not seem to have been affected by the stroke. He posed a challenge to the staff caring for him on the ward. On a number of occasions, he tried to get out of bed, only to end up on the floor, unable to get up. He refused help with toileting, and had to be gently coaxed by his wife. He became quite agitated one night, shouting, 'Who is this in my bed?' and pointing to his left leg that lay motionless by his side.

'He is in clear denial', was his wife's verdict. She had read about denial in a women's magazine. But what manner of denial was this that belied all common sense?

The mention of denial conjures up psychoanalytical concepts according to which denial is a defence mechanism against the awareness of a painful fact despite overwhelming evidence supporting it. A common example is that of a man dismissing a chest pain as indigestion and not seeking emergency treatment in spite of being aware of the seriousness of such a symptom. Denial may result in postponement of the repayment of debts or the lack of acceptance of responsibility for one's actions or in excessive risk-taking behaviour. In such circumstances, denial as a psychological concept has some explanatory power. It was conceptualised as an immature defence by Anna Freud.[12]

Peter could not have been called an immature man before his stroke. He had had a successful career as a structural engineer and was actively involved in a number of clubs and organisations. Moreover, there was clear evidence that the right hemisphere of his brain had suffered a stroke, and the problem had resulted from this event. This association of denial of paralysis with right[13] hemispheric strokes has been recognised by neurologists for more than a century. A famous French neurologist, Joseph Babinski,[14] coined the term *anosognosia* (from Greek, *a* meaning 'without', *nosos*, disease and *gnosis*, knowledge) in 1914 for this presentation. Anosognosia is a broad term and could be used for denial of any type of neurological deficit. The unawareness of one half of the body that Peter showed is referred to as asomatognosia, an unawareness of the body. There are other disorders of awareness such as the denial of blindness, neglect of one side of the visual space and denial of aphasia (severe language disorder), which may be seen as forms of anosognosia. The unawareness in anosognosics persists despite logical arguments and the demonstration of contradictory evidence. They may sometimes come up with fantastic or bizarre explanations, and do not appear to be perturbed when their convictions are challenged. In rare cases, delusion-like ideas may develop. Patients have been described who disclaimed ownership of the limb altogether,[15] and even had a name for the limb as if it belonged to a distinct person. Pathological hatred for the paralytic limb has also been described.

The mechanisms for the production of anosognosia are not known. One theory holds that it is due to the lack of sensory feedback – in the case of Peter, from the left side of the body. We are aware of parts of our bodies because the brain is constantly receiving sensations from the muscles, joints etc. The sensory deficits in the brain may cause the individual to be unable to see or feel the left arm and leg, and there is no proprioceptive or movement related feedback from the limbs. There is some support for this hypothesis, as the lack of awareness may be partially reversed by focusing the patient's attention to the limb in various ways. This cannot, however, be the only explanation. Since anosognosia occurs largely, although not exclusively, with right hemispheric lesions, a right–left hemispheric imbalance has been suggested as another explanation. This has been shown experimentally as well using the Wada Test.[16] In this ingenious technique, a short-acting barbiturate is injected into one carotid artery under radiological guidance so that one hemisphere of the brain is selectively anaesthetised for a short period. The carotid artery supplies blood to the brain, and there is one on either side. Anosognosia is more likely to occur when the injection is on the right side,[17] whereby the right hemisphere is temporarily knocked out. There are a number of hypotheses to explain this observation, none of which is completely satisfactory. These rely on the fact that the left hemisphere is the language repository of the brain, and may have representations from both sides of the body, but depends on information from the right side to maintain a balanced view. Damage to the right hemisphere either leads to the destruction of a large part of the left-sided representation, or produces a right–left discordance, which the left hemisphere compensates by creating a false mental schema. Anosognosia, according to this view, is a failure of the balance between the two hemispheres.[18] Some support for this comes from the observation that the anosognosia can be temporarily reversed by squirting cold water into the left ear canal (caloric stimulation).

Another approach that scientists have taken to explain anosognosia is to examine the role of specific brain regions in our awareness of the body. We know that larger brain lesions are more likely to produce this problem, suggesting that certain specific brain regions may be involved in the neuronal circuits that underlie self-awareness and body perception. Much of the attention has been on the frontal lobes, the large parts of the brain that lie behind the forehead, and in particular the medial prefrontal cortex. This is the region of the frontal lobes that sits on the inside, close to the midline. It has been shown to be active at rest, i.e. its general metabolic rate is high, as if it were working all the time. It is supposed to integrate the various influences that go into forming a concept of 'self' and keep the narrative of the person, thereby helping store the life story of the individual.[19] The medial prefrontal cortex is a complex region, however, and can be divided into dorsal and ventral, or upper and lower, regions with different functions. The relationship to self-representation is therefore complex.

The prefrontal region has also been implicated in the 'theory of mind' or 'mentalising', the cluster of abilities held to be necessary to understand the mental processes of others. While the concept has been around for some time, it was formally discussed by Premack and Woodruff who asked the question, 'Does the chimpanzee have a theory of mind?'[20] Does the chimpanzee know what the other chimpanzee is thinking? Does it realise that others may have similar thoughts and emotions? As human beings, we are quite good at knowing what someone is thinking or feeling, and can relate to the person on her or his terms. Because of the theory of mind, we can attribute feelings, intentions, beliefs and desires to others. A lack of theory of mind has been implicated in the development of autism. Disruption of the medial prefrontal cortex may therefore lead to considerable disturbance in relation to self-representation as well as the representation of others. Whether it explains anosognosia is uncertain. It is important to point out that brain regions do not work in isolation. The prefrontal cortex interacts intimately with the parietal cortex where some of the somatic representation occurs, and it is most likely the disruption of such circuits between different parts of the brain that lies at the heart of body image disturbances.

We of course took this detour to come back to anorexia nervosa with a better understanding of the brain processes that might explain why Anna had a distorted view of her body and why she was not aware of this distortion. My interviews with Anna convinced me of the seriousness of her condition.

I knew that the road to health for her was likely to be a long and arduous one, and this would take the concerted effort of a team of professionals devoted to the treatment of anorexia. Since I did not work in an eating disorders unit, I was not the person to take her on that journey. She was back in the care of my colleague who directed a unit exclusively for the treatment of eating disorders. Her psychiatric assessment did not reveal the presence of any other disorder. A physical examination and blood tests revealed anaemia (low blood count because of deficiency of iron), an electrolyte imbalance (possibly because of vomiting and purging) and abnormal liver function (because of poor nutrition). With her BMI at 15, there was a strong indication to admit her to hospital, which she reluctantly agreed to after her parents presented her with no other option.

Once in hospital, the treatment strategy was like well-oiled machinery. The psychiatrist, nurses, social worker and psychologist had well-defined roles. Each of them worked to establish a relationship with Anna. She was given a great deal of education on anorexia. The psychologist worked on some motivational techniques to improve her cooperation and enhance her motivation to change. She was required to keep a food diary for the first few days. A meeting was then held to plan goals for her treatment in the short term, to be reviewed in a week. A diet plan was agreed upon with the help of the dietician. She was required to eat three regularly spaced meals per day, keep a food diary of all other foods eaten, eat in the presence of nurses and remain with them for at least one hour after meals. This was because anorexia patients, while otherwise highly moral, are known to cheat when it comes to food, and many have a strong urge to induce vomiting after their meals. She was told that she would be discharged from hospital only when her weight was in the normal BMI range and she was showing evidence that normal eating patterns had been restored. Medication was discussed with her, and she was started on olanzapine, an anti-psychotic drug that is known to also increase appetite and cause weight gain. While she was not considered to be psychotic, it was hoped that the drug would dent the conviction with which she held the belief that her body was fat.

Anna took three months to gain the target weight. There were many struggles on the way, including periods when she refused to eat and her privileges had to be taken away. The psychiatrist and psychologists worked together to keep her motivated and engaged. They also attempted to modify her thinking through cognitive behaviour therapy. She had to be taught how to challenge her disordered thoughts about eating and weight. A greater mindfulness of her own thoughts was required. She was beginning to ask herself questions in relation to her thoughts: does this thought help me achieve my goals? What is the worst that can happen if this thought is true? How likely is this outcome? How will I cope with the worst possible outcome? Am I applying the same standards to myself as I apply to others? Is there another way I can think about this? Am I being too negative? Can this be phrased differently?

After discharge from hospital, Anna continued to see her psychiatrist. He kept a close eye on her eating habits and her weight. He engaged her in therapy to foster healthy beliefs about her body weight and shape. There were a number of issues in relation to her low self-esteem, guilt and shame, and poor interpersonal relationships, all of which needed attention. Since Anna was still living at home, her family was included in the treatment. Her olanzapine was gradually stopped more than three months after discharge. Her periods returned after six months, and the baby hair was gone.

I saw Anna two years later. She was an attractive young woman who had gained weight and was now in the low normal range of BMI. She had a much healthier perception of herself, although there were days when she still struggled with the image in the mirror and the food on her plate. She had learnt to regard her weight and body image as a disorder that needed treatment, and I considered that to be a major breakthrough. She recognised that most people considered her to be thin. She resumed her university degree and was happy with her performance. She had had a boyfriend for six months. She continued to see her psychiatrist once every fortnight, and was fearful of a relapse if she discontinued her treatment. I asked her to draw an image of herself on a blank piece of paper. She produced a fairly accurate impression, without the distortion that was so remarkable in the first interview.

Yet I knew that it was going to be a long road for her. Thankfully, she was showing the correct signs of improvement. Most patients of anorexia eventually do improve and often look back with amazement that their perceptions could have been so erroneous. It is reassuring that the disordered brain has within it the capacity to recover when provided with the right environment. Anorexia provides a window into the 'new' neuroscience in which the psychological and neurobiological interweave. It illustrates how the environment can act on the brain to produce changes that in turn influence the environment the individual creates. The message to young people is: beware this whirlpool!

6

The dead homunculus

The entire period of human evolutionary existence can be viewed as the age of the frontal lobe.

Tilney, *The Brain from Ape to Man*[1]

I had decided to see Stephen somewhat reluctantly. The story Dr Sabiosky – his family doctor and my friend – related in his referral letter seemed ordinary: a head-injured young man who was suing for compensation. Predictable, I thought. Multiple symptoms laced with a tinge of neurosis, it must be! I must confess to a certain bias against such cases. Medico-legal matters bore me, with their endless hours in court on legal battles with little relevance to medicine, and even less understanding of it. The patient is playing a dual act during the examination, a court performance in the clinic, with the invisible but ever-present audience influencing every move. 'No', I would ordinarily say, but I agreed to see him to give an opinion as Dr Sabiosky appeared to be struggling with his mangement. My consultations with Stephen extended to many sessions, which also involved interviewing his family and many interviews with his ex-girlfriend, who appeared to still care for him a great deal. It also included one admission to our ward for observation, and attempts to help Stephen with his problems.

If first impressions can influence one's judgment, my biases were only reinforced: long hair done crudely in a ponytail with an elastic band. A gold ring in the left ear! But the smile on the face was charming, and he sat upright with a confidence that softened me. 'He should be anxious', I thought, 'for my opinion may influence the outcome of his case.' No, he seemed relaxed, and not in awe – even somewhat familiar – a sort of 'matey' attitude so peculiarly Australian. He picked up a pen from my desk and began playing with it, proceeding to draw something on his hand I could not see.

'Can I see what you are drawing?' I asked.

'It's nothing, doc. You mind if I call you doc ... what is it now, Doctor ... er ... Sachdev? I've got it right, I hope?' I nodded, drawing his attention again to his hand on which I could now see a doodle.

'Oh yes, the drawing! I'm no artist. Well, no, not this sort of artist. I'm a performer. I sing and play in a band. At least, I used to until the accident.' He tapped his fingers on the desk, playing a mock piano. Actions seemed to flow out of him as easily as words, and both were telling the same story. He was a genuine person, I thought.

I went through the details of his accident – which happened three years ago – with him, not for the sake of further information (the account was already available to me from his previous doctors) but to get an idea of his recollection of the events. The memory deficit was consistent with earlier descriptions: little recollection of events for a few hours before the accident (the so-called retrograde amnesia), and a blank slate for more than a week after (anterograde amnesia). The injury had been quite severe, with an extensive fracture of the head and damage to the frontal and temporal lobes easily seen on a CT brain scan. The first two weeks had been agonising, and it seemed likely that the Stephen who emerged would be encumbered in a number of ways. But the reparative powers of the human brain are remarkable indeed. It sustains injury, falters for a while, then restores much that has been lost. And this is despite the fact that the generation of new cells is limited in the brain to a few regions only, and its significance in brain repair is uncertain. The brain must rearrange itself, in a way. Nature, being practical, is more concerned with function. And is not the preservation of function the greater need? Stephen's doctors had watched his memory take the first few wobbly steps and gradually walk quite unaided. Two years on, the neuropsychologist testing him could find no problem with his memory with the usual bag of neuropsychological tests. And he did equally well on tests of the frontal lobe, the part of the brain responsible for higher mental functions, and indeed our personality and intelligence. Nature had seemingly repaired, or rather overcome, most of the damage.

Or had it? Stephen's life had changed. To a casual observer, he seemed quite normal. He had always been the 'odd one out' of the family. While his brothers had emulated their father and made strides in academia, he had mixed with the fringe of society, searching for a career in entertaining. The promised chart-popping record never arrived, but small scandals came with enough regularity to drive his usually tolerant parents to total non-involvement with their prodigal son. They did not approve of his life before the accident, but recognised the fact that all his actions were of his own choosing – he had been in good control of his life. Now he was a different man, a post-accident Stephen who was pushed around by stimuli from within and without. All 'impulse and echo', as his father put it.

The impulse struck me without warning, although warned I should have been. I asked him about his financial situation and he laughed – not a cynical laugh that hides contempt, but a hilarious laugh, soon becoming a hysteric, turning me immediately into an observer of a clever mimic. The laughter persisted for some time, and seemed interminable. When quiet descended, he showed no sign that anything inappropriate had happened; no apology for such a dramatic release was forth-coming. It happened once again a few minutes later, this time a well of tears on the mention of a recently departed female friend. The show was intense, but the storm seemed to occur on the surface, with no deeper stirrings. Like a cyclone, it came with little warning and passed quickly. The story narrated by his relatives was similar. The pre-accident Stephen had been intense and deep, a man who felt his passion. The post-accident Stephen (for there were two Stephens, one before and one after the accident) wore his emotions on his sleeve, but they did not seem to stir his heart. What could have gone wrong in the brain to cause this?

Imagine a little man, a homunculus[2] sitting in the front of the brain, controlling the traffic, letting some emotions pass, stopping them when their time had run out, testing them for their reasonableness and their need, acting as both policeman and judge. This little man seemed to have lost his balance in Stephen's brain, his proper perspective, his ability to judge what was right. Had he been KO'd by the head injury? Was Stephen suffering from the 'dead homunculus syndrome'?

The two brief episodes in my office signalled the chaos his

emotions were creating in his life. His former female friend illustrated this rather vividly. 'Previously, he was faithful, and mostly kind, but furious when he was offended. And, he was full of oomph and verve ... and a certain tenacity.' And now, she said, 'He snarls and gnashes his teeth at the slightest provocation. He is loving at times, but then attacks me like a madman. I could not live with him any more.' His poorly controlled anger led him into brawls in which his fury did not terminate until he was exhausted. There were two charges of serious bodily harm awaiting trial. Anyone who had witnessed one of his episodes avoided him. The friend's description was reminiscent of that by Hermann Boerhaave, who first provided evidence of a brain lesion producing uncontrolled aggression in 1715, using the example of a rabid dog. Boerhaave (1668–1738),[3] the founder of Dutch medicine, was one of the greatest clinical teachers of his time in the Hippocratic tradition. We owe him some of the earliest insights into the relationship between brain and behaviour. His most unusual case was the 'walking experimental preparation', a beggar who roamed the streets of Paris using his calvarium, the removed cap of his skull, as his begging bowl. For a 'small trifle of money', he would permit experiments to be conducted in which the dura mater (the thick membrane covering the brain) could be pressed by the experimenter. What better subject for a great clinician-experimenter!

Stephen was aware of his loss of control. 'It comes on like lightning ... too quickly ... much before I can do anything about it. And, it takes over. I know I do crazy things – break my furniture, even hit my girlfriend – but I cannot control myself ... It can take me an hour or more to feel calm again

... I am exhausted at the end of it all ... I wish you would give me a pill to control my temper.' The well-known psychiatrist G. A. Kaplan, as early as 1899, recognised the features of such outbursts, likening the phenomenon to a 'pure psychic reflex', as if the intermediating homunculus was dead. He had himself escaped a homicidal attack and remembered the attacker vividly: 'his eyes darkened and his moustache bristled'. His descriptions of such outbursts are quite evocative:[4]

> Following the most trivial and most impersonal causes, there is the effect of rage with its motor accompaniments. There may be the most grotesque gesticulations, excessive movements of the face, and a quick, sharp explosiveness of speech; there may be cursing and outbreaks of violence which are often directed towards things; there may or may not be amnesia for these events afterwards. These outbursts may terminate in an epileptic fit. There is an excess in the reaction with inadequate adaptation to the situation which is so remote from a well considered and purposeful act that it approaches a pure psychic reflex.

Monroe, in 1974, called this feature 'episodic dyscontrol': 'an interruption in the lifestyle and life flow of the individual, involving either a single act or short series of acts with a single intention ...'[5] This term has had a chequered career, with Vernon Mark, a Boston neurosurgeon, and Frank Ervin, a Californian psychiatrist, making it notorious with their 1970 book, *Violence and the Brain*, in which they suggested that all violent behaviour had a basis in brain pathology and should possibly be treated with brain surgery.[6] Monroe's dyscontrol patients were different from Stephen in some ways, the most important of which was their abnormality on EEG, a recording of the electrical activity of the brain. Monroe regarded these outbursts as being equivalent to seizures or epilepsy, the implication being that the individual was afflicted with the problem that was not of his or her making. Such behaviour, even when destructive, warranted understanding by society: it should be dealt with from a medical and not a criminal perspective. Stephen's EEG was entirely normal, even, as on one occasion, soon after an aggressive outburst. This was evidence that the outburst was not an epileptic seizure, but of course the aggression still stemmed from a brain abnormality.

Stephen's dyscontrol went further than his aggression, or his laughter, or even his tears. He showed little restraint in describing his physical and sexual prowess to the nurses who attended to him on the ward, and invited one of them to bed, only to be mildly rebuked. His former girlfriend had been concerned about his sexual disinhibition. He had become disinhibited, tending to kiss her passionately in public places and touching her awkwardly and suggestively. In the initial period after the head injury, he made frequent requests for sexual intercourse, only to discover each time that he was impotent.

He reminded me of a famous case in the literature: a 39-year-old New York stockbroker described by Brickner in the 1930s after he had much of both frontal lobes removed because of a large meningioma (a tumour of the brain originating from the meningeal membranes that cover the brain).[7] Like Stephen, A. was impotent but loved to talk about his sexual exploits, mixing fact with fantasy until he himself no longer knew the difference. A. has a special place in the history of psychiatry because of the impression he created on Egaz Moniz,[8] the pioneer of psychosurgery. Moniz was so impressed by the fact that A. had retained most of his higher faculties after such extensive lesions of the frontal lobes, and had also joined the 'happiness cult',[9] that he tested the possibility that frontal lobe surgery may be a treatment for severe psychiatric disorders. The 'happiness cult' had been earlier suggested by the American neuroscientist Jacobsen who performed frontal lobe surgery on monkeys to note their subsequent behaviour. Both Stephen and A. were 'witty', but the jokes were at other people's expense. When the tables were turned, Stephen responded with anger and accusation. The jocularity was in reality facetiousness; the wit was *witzelsucht* (from German: *witzel(ei)* meaning pun or joke, and *sucht* meaning addiction or yearning). I now had doubts about Stephen's genuineness.

Stephen made me aware, like no other patient, of the passions hidden in the human soul. Freud was probably observing the same passions when he recognised the id. Alternatively, one could call it the primitive part of the brain, the animal hiding inside our heads whose fangs have not been pulled, merely trimmed, by culture. The cloak of civilisation had been partially shed by his head injury, and what emerged was frightening. Was the cloak so thin, human-ness so fragile, civilisation no more than the consequence of a few layers of neurones in the front of the brain whose removal did not even affect intelligence? There must be a greater mystery to these so-called frontal lobes than had been revealed, I thought to myself, or do we make too much of our human nature?[10]

I had seen the impulses, but what of the echoes? They were far less obvious, not declaring themselves with the intensity of the emotions or the drama of the violence. In their subtlety lay their impact, however, for it was difficult to comprehend the reach of their reverberations. His behaviour echoed his environment or his passion, like a tiny boat adrift in a mighty ocean. 'He munched all day with little awareness of his meals. I reminded him to save some appetite for the meal, and he usually promised, and yet the next time he saw a packet of chips, or an apple in the basket, and off he went once more,' his ex-girlfriend explained. 'He just could not keep himself from it … The feeling I got was that he could not direct himself.' Life for him had become like that – driven by stimulus. He would embarrass her by staring at any young woman who passed by, and would even call out to her. 'He was never a cautious man, but always was aware of his self-interest and guarded it. Now it is different. It is gratification he wants … He does not know when it hurts him. He is his own worst enemy.'

He was an intelligent man, 'above average in his intellectual abilities' as our clinical psychologist put it. The National Adult Reading Test (NART)[11] and Wechsler's tests of intelligence showed that he still performed at about the same as the estimated level before the accident in his overall 'intelligence'. But what good was his intelligence to him if he could not stop himself from acting inappropriately at every step? The 'intelligence tests' presumably did not measure the social corpuscles, his ability to conduct himself in society. He had a good knowledge of etiquette, but when it came to dressing himself, the first article within reach in his cupboard was a good enough apparel. His dress was not a product of poverty, or an attempt at casualness, but a reflection of disorganisation. It seemed that the clothes, rather than the wearer, decided whose turn it was to be worn. Neatness and cleanliness were further casualties, which ended in chaos if a friend or his mother did not intervene. He had returned to playing in the band, but his friends had gently persuaded him that he needed some more time to settle back into his life. His mother was aware of the difficulties: 'He has lost that flexibility that a musician needs. He can follow the score all right, but now and again the same note repeats itself, as if the record got stuck. There are times when he is expected to follow on from another player but he tends to repeat what has already been played. It does not happen very often, but even one such occurrence can ruin a performance ... He, of course, would not acknowledge it.' Stephen still boasted of his musical talent, and when reminded that he had not written anything since his accident, he merely shrugged it off. 'I have to seriously get back into a band before the inspiration comes,' he explained.

I was now beginning to understand the real problems this young man faced when on the surface, and on 'intelligence' tests, he passed for normal. I went back to the published literature to make more sense of this puzzle, and once again Professor Alexander Luria,[12] the great Russian neuropsychologist, came to the rescue. Luria was a keen observer of behaviour, and his study material was the many Russian veterans who had received head injuries in battle. One of his patients went to the railway station and took the first available train, with little regard for his destination. Another patient would press his bedside button whenever he saw it, even though there was never a need to summon the nurse. Luria called it reflexive behaviour, a mechanical action occurring on a cue, with little need to presuppose an intervening entity such as the mind or will. Professor Lhermitte, of the Salpêtrière in Paris, calls it the environmental dependency syndrome, with the patient's actions being determined not by his 'will' but rather by the exigencies of the environment. It was suggested to Lhermitte's patient, on his trip to the professor's apartment (which was arranged as part of an experiment), that he was in a museum, and he immediately started to methodically examine the paintings. When he found a painting on the floor, and some nails and a hammer nearby, he proceeded to hang the painting in the vacant spot on the wall. Further on in his exploration of the apartment, he encountered a bed with the top sheet turned back. He immediately began to undress, got into the bed, pulled the sheet up to his neck and prepared to sleep.

I was reminded of my earlier encounter with Stephen when he had picked up my pen to draw with it. Was he exhibiting the same so-called utilisation behaviour, in which he grasped and used any object presented to him irrespective of need? Was his mind a ping-pong ball, changing direction with every stroke from outside? When Stephen was admitted to the neuropsychiatry ward for observation, I decided to test it using Professor Lhermitte's clinical techniques.

The first step was to examine for imitation behaviour. In my next session with him I equipped myself with a range of objects to aid me. During the course of the interview, I purposely performed a few gestures to see if he copied any. I bent my head forwards and rested my chin on my hand, but this did not seem to have any effect on him. I slapped my thigh with my hand but again with no success. But when I tapped the table with my hand, he repeated my action. A few minutes later, I did it again, and again it was repeated. I crossed my legs, and so did he. I was now beginning to be convinced that this was not a coincidence. I had previously placed two sheets of paper and two envelopes on the desk, within easy reach of both of us. I took one sheet of paper, folded it carefully and put it in the envelope. I could observe his hand crawl toward the paper, but he did not take it. Getting even more dramatic, I made a military salute. He looked puzzled, examined his hand but did not copy me. I began to hum. He was amused but did not join me. I picked up a comb from the desk and ran it through my hair with seriousness. Although another comb lay within his reach, he did not pick it, but his hand went up to brush his hair. I then picked up a pen and proceeded to write a sentence. So did he, except that he just scribbled and did not write anything meaningful.

Was Stephen imitating other people's actions in real life as well? His parents had noticed that he would join them in certain activities when he was clearly not needed. His mother was annoyed at his 'habit' of standing beside her and fiddling with the pans when she was cooking. When queried about something, he had a tendency to repeat the question, a 'habit' the pre-accident Stephen again did not have. His mother provided an example:

'When will you be joining us in the restaurant, Stephen?'

'When will I be joining you? About seven o'clock.'

Not unusual if it happened occasionally, or if you had not known Stephen before the change! He was apparently not aware of this behaviour. I drew his attention to our earlier interview, and again he was not aware that he had repeated anything I had done. 'I just felt like doing all those things,' he remarked. He did not consider any need for an explanation.

For my next session with him, I put some medical instruments on my desk. I had asked my secretary to ring as soon as he came through so that I could pretend to be attending to the call. He picked up the reflex hammer and tapped his arms with it for a while. He then proceeded to tap his knees, trying to elicit a reflex in the manner he was surely familiar with, having been subjected to a number of neurological examinations. As my talk with my secretary continued, he put the hammer down and picked up the tongue depressor, put it into his mouth and pressed his tongue with it. I finished my conversation and looked at him questioningly. 'Sorry, doc, I was playing with your instruments. I hope you don't mind.' Without answering him, I got up from my chair and proceeded towards the door. He followed me out of the room and into the small back garden. I sat on the bench outside, and he came and sat beside me. No word had been exchanged between us. I got up to go back to the office, and he followed me once more. The rest of the session continued in the office.

During the course of his stay in the ward, another opportunity presented itself: a pre-Christmas luncheon to which patients and staff were invited. Stephen made no contribution to the preparation of the meal or the decorations that go with it. 'He lacks all interest,' remarked one of the nurses. 'All the other patients volunteered to help.' At mealtime, however, his behaviour was quite different. He was playing the host, pouring drinks for everybody, handing out plates and encouraging everybody to take more food, including myself. Stephen as the insistent host was a picture of him I had not anticipated.

I decided to send him for a magnetic resonance imaging (MRI)[13] brain scan to get more detailed information on the extent of his brain damage. The result was not surprising. There was extensive damage to both frontal lobes – the parts of the brain that project out in front and seem to distinguish, by their size, us humans from our animal ancestors – in particular the parts above the eye sockets, with the right lobe being more affected. The right temporal lobe was also damaged.

Had I been able to synthesise a cohesive whole that this young man represented? Who and what made up the real Stephen? Was he a chameleon who adopted the colour of his environs? A ping-pong ball, as I already said; or is the correct appellation 'Hume's billiard ball', after the eighteenth-century philosopher David Hume … or a stimulus-bound automaton … a ship without a captain? And sometimes a spluttering, boiling cauldron or a melting figure of wax. He was a musician with a few broken strings, which had been tightened nevertheless … an artist whose creativity was dead, a lover whose passion had lost tenderness and feeling. He was all these things at different times, but the thread that linked these miniature Stephens had snapped. The real Stephen had, in fact, splintered into a thousand pieces. There was no Stephen to say 'no', and similarly no-one to say 'not yet'. One could call this lack of inhibition, or the presence of 'imitation' and 'utilisation' behaviour, but this missed the point. To analyse pathology in behaviour, one has to presuppose the presence of a person. I was still searching for this person in the man I saw before me.

For Immanuel Kant, 'a person is a subject who is responsible for his actions'. The imitating, utilising, environmentally dependent Stephen was not, therefore, a Kantian person. On two counts he failed: autonomy and responsibility for actions, which, to my mind, remain the essence of personhood. As Sir

Karl Popper conjectures in the book *The Self and Its Brain*: 'The self is not a "pure ego", that is, a mere subject. Rather, it is incredibly rich. Like a pilot, it observes and takes action at the same time. It is acting and suffering, recalling the past and planning and programming the future; expecting and disposing … And all this closely interacts with the tremendous activity that goes on in the brain.'[14]

The pilot in Stephen's brain was having tremendous difficulty with the activity that went on in it. Would it be right to say that Stephen had lost his 'free will', at least partially? Was he responsible for attacking his girlfriend and hurting her feelings? Was it he, again, playing with my instruments and acting the host at the table? In some ways it was right to say so. He was aware of what he was doing, acknowledged it, knew that it might be considered inappropriate behaviour by some (without this influencing his actions) and even apologised for it on occasion. But could he have stopped himself? Put in the same situation, and advised to behave differently, would he have demonstrated an ability to choose? And, if yes, was his choice flexible? Or was he driven inexorably by brute forces deep within the layers of his brain? Had his behaviour become mechanical – the product of a 'mindless' automaton – so that he was the 'mere plaything of external forces', as Robert Nozick would say?[15] To some extent it had; the impulses and echoes that he manifested were not the products of a rational, responsible person. Images of the external words made an impression on his mind, and found direct expression in his actions – in a kind of a short circuit. A supervisory system that would normally assess and assimilate the impressions was missing.[16] The same happened to powerful passions that were aroused within. Yet, if he was not responsible for these, was he diminished as a person? Was he less than human because of his actions?

Puzzled by all these questions that welled up in my mind, I resorted to a simple psychiatrist's trick: I threw them back at Stephen for his answers. He was aware of his emotionality, his impulsiveness. 'But in a way I have always been that way,' he said. 'It was one reason my family never liked me. I always felt that it was the more natural way of being ... I was living life to the full ... I know that recently it has become a problem for me ... perhaps the accident has sent me around the bend a bit, but I still would rather be impulsive than straight and stuffy like my brothers.' What of his imitation behaviour? He hadn't noticed it. 'I, of course, have a bit of a performer in me ...' He acknowledged full responsibility for his actions. He felt like a whole person. By his account, there was nothing the matter with him except that people found him difficult to get on with and the accident had ruined his career and almost killed him.

Stephen was not 'psychological', not your perfect self-watcher, who asked questions of himself. He had been like this even before the accident. The head injury had surely done something to him. Could it have simply exaggerated the 'deficiencies' (or his strengths, depending upon who was talking) in his personality that already existed? Were we still seeing the real Stephen, perhaps a little blown up and larger than life? Could we argue that his frontal lobes had always been somewhat dysfunctional? Was the pre-accident Stephen similarly diminished by biology, only less so? Can we say the same about all people who are impulsive, or fickle, or irrational, or temperamental?

I think that this line of thinking could be a trap for the

unwary. Yes, frontal lobe functioning is equated with reason and judgment and perhaps free will. Yes, frontal lobe damage produces a loss of these qualities. Yes, again, these qualities are considered to be the ones that immediately separate man from beast. But these qualities vary from person to person. Where do we draw the line? At what stage, on the continuum of these qualities, does a person lose his or her personhood? Absolute free will is a myth even existential philosophers shy away from. How much more of free will needs to be destroyed before a man becomes a wasp, a *Sphex ichneumoneus* of Douglas Hofstadter's description,[17] whose painfully complex routine is but the result of a hard-wired program? If Stephen had emerged from the accident even more impulsive, even more environmentally dependent, would he have been even more waspish? The 'intelligent' robots would have us believe so even though they have no way of packing passion into their silicon bodies. For me Stephen remained human … a whole person … admittedly, weak and impulsive – yes, less than perfect, but a human being nevertheless. My analytical mind had led me into a thought abyss, much like Dennett's snake that started swallowing its tail until it had swallowed itself completely. As soon as I suspended my critical judgment and met Stephen on a human plane, I could feel for – and indeed with – him. I did not approve of his behaviour, but I was convinced that as long as there was behavioural output from this individual, he remained a person. My soul could touch his, and that was my surest test of his personhood.

Stephen's mimicry made me think about another recent discovery in neuroscience that has caused a great deal of excitement: that of the mirror neuron system. Scientists have

always wondered why we imitate others. Why is it that watching someone yawn has an infectious quality about it? Why do
our feet start tapping when we watching those twisting legs
on the dance floor or listen to the beat of Panjabi bhangra
music? When watching Roger Federer deliver his lethal back-
hand, you may sometimes notice your own arm performing a
mock swing. There must be the seeds of mimicry in our brains.
A mother instinctively knows this when she makes babbling
sounds in front of her baby and pokes out her tongue at the
little one. Mirror neurons offer such a rich basis for explaining
many aspects of human behaviour that they deserve further
discussion.

Neuroscientists at the University of Parma in Italy were-
taken by surprise when they came upon the possible neural
basis of such mimicry. The three scientists, Giacomo Rizzolatti, Vittorio Gallese and Leonardo Fogassi, were recording the
electrical activity in single neurons in the frontal lobe of a
monkey as it performed certain actions. They had noted that a
particular set of neurons fired whenever the monkey reached
out to pick a raisin. These neurons lie in the back part of the
frontal lobes, labelled area F5, adjacent to neurons that are
involved in integrating sensory and motor information in relation to grasping. One day, Fogassi walked into the room and
casually picked up a raisin. As the monkey watched him do this
act, the same neuron in the monkey's brain started firing as if it
was performing the grasping act itself. Fogassi was amazed by
this and repeated the experiment many times, grasping different objects, or moving his hand without grasping, taking the
food to his mouth or to his side, and performing other movements. The scientists discovered that a set of neurons was active

when the monkey performed reaching, grasping and manipulating tasks or watched these tasks being performed by another monkey or human. They dubbed these the mirror neurons. They discovered another area of the brain in the parietal lobe that was intimately connected to this system. The parietal area was the sensory (or input) area of this system, whereas the frontal region was the motor (or output) area, comprising the frontoparietal motor neuron system.[18]

Evidence for a mirror neuron system in humans that resembles one seen in monkeys has come from imaging studies, especially those using functional magnetic resonance imaging (fMRI). Another region in the temporal lobe is important in providing higher-order visual input to the mirror neuron system, and these three areas may be considered to be the core circuit for imitation. These mirror neurons are present from birth and may play a major role in the development of social behaviour as well as language. Jean Piaget was struck by the fact that his infant child poked out his tongue in imitation. In early life, children do mirror-image imitation: when the child sees a left hand being raised, it raises its right hand. Neuroimaging studies have shown that such mirror-image imitation produces a greater response in the mirror neurons than an anatomically correct imitation, suggesting that imitation may be crucial for the development of behaviour. What is even more interesting is that children tend to imitate the goal of the action they observe rather than the precise movements. It is this imitation that builds their repertoire of socially appropriate actions and may contribute to the social networks they generate.

Of course, as we grow, the activity of mirror neurons must be kept in check so that imitative behaviour is not socially disruptive. Was this Stephen's failing? Had his brain injury allowed his mirror neurons to work with impunity? The echoes were being generated by these nerve cells, and the activity was flowing out unhindered. His utilisation behaviour might have a similar explanation: the sight of an object generated a response in the mirror neuron system for a goal-directed action using that object. This should normally have been suppressed by a well-functioning frontal lobe that was judging the appropriateness of the action. It was this lack of normal suppression that was characteristically aberrant in his behaviour. Had Stephen been a mimic on the stage, he would have generated roars of laughter in the audience. The mimicry of a comedian strikes a chord with the onlookers who can see both the sense and the nonsense in the actions. Stephen failed to realise that the Shakespearean dictum 'All the world's a stage, and all the men and women merely players ...' was not to be taken literally.

The mirror neuron system may be important for the acquisition of language. When we hear someone speak, there is activity not only in those parts of the brain that deal with reception of speech and analysis of language, but also in the brain region in the frontal lobe responsible for the production of speech – the so-called Broca's area. If this activity is suppressed using a magnetic pulse, imitation is impaired, suggesting that this part is important for imitation of speech. It might explain the importance of the 'baby talk' a mother engages in and the ease with which a child picks up a language.[19]

Most importantly for humans, the mirror neurons play an important role in socialisation. Humans imitate each other in social interaction – they copy facial expressions and body postures – and the more they imitate, the more empathic they tend to be.[20] Imagine going to a psychiatrist who sits in front of you and periodically repeats the questions: 'Can you tell me a little more?' 'That must have felt terrible!' 'Yes, go on!' 'Can you say that again?' and so on, but shows no change of facial expression, intonation or posture. He does not bend forward when you are distressed, does not show surprise when you mention the betrayal you suffered from a close friend, and does not offer you a tissue if you break down in tears. Would you go back to such a psychiatrist? This psychiatrist does not recognise the value of imitation – he may as well be a robot. No wonder robots have proven not to be effective psychotherapists even though they can be programmed to say the right thing most of the time!

Bruno Wicker of the University of the Mediterranean in Marseilles published an interesting study in which he imaged the brains of individuals who either felt disgusted themselves (from seeing a disgusting stimulus) or watched other people who had an expression of disgust.[21] Both produced similar activity in a brain region called the insula, which is linked to the limbic system (the part of the brain dealing with emotion) and the mirror neuron system. The mirror neurons are therefore important for emotional contagion – the fact that the moment you walk into a room in which everyone is happy has an uplifting effect on the mood, and sitting next to a depressed person can wear you down heavily. Activity in this system may be the reason we can read other people's emotions so well, and why Stephen was so hopeless in judging other people's responses accurately. He could not appreciate that his behaviour was causing embarrassment to his family and friends. The overactivity in his mirror neuron system had possibly led to poor or abnormal functioning of the network linking this system with the limbic system as well as the frontal executive system.

This brings us to the role of mirror neurons in the theory of mind. I will discuss this as it relates to Stephen in a different sort of way. Human beings have the ability to attribute mental states to others and equate these with their own mental states. We can judge what someone else is thinking or wants to do, and attribute an intention to their actions. It seems that mirror neurons may play a part in this. These neurons respond differently to grasping action depending upon what was intended – whether the grasp of a cup was, for example for drinking or for cleaning up.[22] They also distinguish between an individual working at a computer from two persons conversing with each other.

Not surprisingly, there has been considerable interest in the study of the mirror neuron system in autism, a disorder of brain development in which a child grows up with considerable problems in social interaction and communication. Autistic children have a fundamental problem in relating to other people. Human infants are able to imitate the facial and hand gestures of others, and by the age of one year, they have proactive goal-directed eye movements, suggesting that they can predict the actions of others. Autistic children are deficient in this ability, which makes it difficult for them to appreciate the mental state of others and develop representations of their intentions. This leads to a great difficulty in relating with others, so that the autistic individual is most uncomfortable when confronted with situations in which they have to deal with people. In fact, they prefer animals or animate objects that do not require a similar degree of mentalising.

Stephen, of course, did not have this problem, but perhaps his problem was the reverse. His overactive mirror neurons attributed mental states to others when none existed, or over-attributed intention. The consequence was a suspiciousness or paranoia that, although not delusional, was difficult for others to accept. His partner had borne the brunt of his paranoid rage. I wish I had a method by which I could switch off his overactive mirror neurons.

I continued to see Stephen over the next year. While he was not seeking treatment for his behavioural change, his family was keen that medications be tried to dampen down his aggressiveness and impulsivity. There were a limited number of drugs for this purpose in my bag, and I was pessimistic about their effectiveness. I persuaded Stephen to take fluoxetine (Prozac), a drug to increase serotonin levels in the brain. He suffered from nausea and headache from the drug, but it appeared to have little effect on his behaviour. He went on to try a number of other drugs, which included mood stablisiers and antipsychotics. I was not convinced that the benefit to Stephen outweighed the adverse effects from the drugs, and he complained bitterly about the medication whenever we met. Eventually, I came to an empirical conclusion that the drugs had not worked, and he was pleased to be off all medication.

His regular visits to see me were of some assistance. We discussed various incidents in his life, his 'failings' as we began to call them. This served a dual purpose: some habitual triggers for his exasperating behaviour were identified, and he was repeatedly reminded of what the appropriate behaviour should have been and how he could have achieved it. I was serving as a surrogate frontal lobe, with the limitation that I could not be with him every moment of his life. This manner of treatment is frustrating for both therapist and patient, as little evidence of change can be mustered from week to week. Over a longer period, the plasticity of the brain does manifest itself and patience is rewarded. I offered to refer him to a rehabilitation specialist, but he declined.

A few months into this treatment, he won his case for compensation, but the payout, although substantial, did not change his life as dramatically as he had hoped. Two more women came into his life and departed disappointed. His parents kept a close watch on him, maintaining his finances and acting as the organising parts of his brain, more out of obligation than devotion and care. He continued to 'live' life, aware that it was his life and he was responsible for it. The money from his compensation payout was securely invested by a public guardian, and regular amounts given to him to meet his genuine needs but not his extravagance. A cocoon had gradually been woven around him – a soft shield that did not bruise his hands when he knocked too hard, as he was prone to do. He would falter now and again, but the damage to his frontal lobes had also done that magical thing – his despair did not turn into a depression, and negative feelings slid just as smoothly through his slippery mind as the positive ones. Life continued to be a roller-coaster ride for both him and his loved ones, and I had just helped secure the safety harness a bit tighter. I hoped that time would gradually dampen the turbulence further.

7

Serotonin's seductive song

Do you know what 'the English vice' really is? Not flagellation,
not pederasty – whatever the French believe it to be. It's our refusal
to admit our emotions. We think they demean us, I suppose.

Terence Rattigan (1911–77), *In Praise of Love* (1973)

'I cannot believe that a drug can change the way I feel' was the incredulous response of Richard when I diagnosed him with depression and recommended medication.

I was used to this reaction from patients. Our emotions are deeply personal. We like to think that the warm glow of love is a blessing that transcends the fetters of language, let alone the unromantic flow of chemicals in the brain. My happiness at my daughter's minor medal in the school swimming competition could not be captured within the amok molecules of dopamine. Depressed patients feel a deep pain within their minds and relate it to the tribulations of their existence. They realise that the psychiatrist cannot change their life's circumstances or its history. But they bear a hope that he will help them find that elusive path that bypasses the pain and distress. They are looking for a 'terrain specialist', as one of my colleagues put it. They want to be better able to navigate the wilderness of the emotional landscape, yet sometimes recoil with horror at the thought that someone would try to change the landscape itself to make it more readily negotiable.

Richard had come to me with a grave problem. He was no longer able to feel the normal range of emotions that he previously took for granted. He told me that his daughter topped her grade at school, and he felt not a twinge of happiness. The sight of his baby boy used to fill him with joy and excitement. He now turned away, paralysed in his emotions. He could not understand what had happened to him.

Richard was a lawyer whose wife and family doctor had persuaded him to see me. He had done so reluctantly, repudiating his English heritage of the stiff upper lip. There was nothing wrong with his life, as far as his wife Anne could tell. 'I love him dearly, and we have two wonderful children,' she explained. 'His career is going well – or so everyone thinks! I have spoken to one of his colleagues to find out whether there was a problem at work. The colleague did say he had noticed that Richard was not as engaged as before, but he considered this to be Richard's personal affair. Nothing else has happened, as far as I can tell. I can't understand why he should be depressed.'

I had diagnosed Richard to be suffering from endogenous depression. The word 'endogenous' implied that the depression had come from within – there was no major stress in his life that was feeding it. His Depression was with a capital 'D' – a disorder, a diagnosis, and not an exaggerated 'sadness' we experience when we suffer a loss or a setback. Its manifestations clearly proved my point. He told me that everything was moving 'swimmingly' until about three months ago when he started noticing problems with his sleep. Nothing dramatic had happened to upset him. He had had an argument at work, and he was working on a difficult case, but there was nothing outstanding about this – these events were the run-of-the-mill problems he faced in his job. Then the mornings became increasingly difficult. He would wake up before sunrise – often at 4 a.m. – and feel a sense of agitation. He stayed in bed and moved very little so as not to disturb his wife. However hard he tried, the sleep appeared to have vanished from his eyes. The mind would then fill up with all sorts of thoughts – usually worrying ones. 'This would go wrong, that would happen, my mother's health, whether my wife was happy with me …' The next few hours were the most miserable part of the day for him. Yet it would be very difficult for Anne to get him out of bed and ready for work. The challenges awaiting him at work no longer provided the motivation to hurry along. He would often be running late and 'You could see from his face that he did not want to go,' Anne added.

It happened gradually – it was difficult to pinpoint a day when he changed. The world had taken on a different hue – a decided grey, as he put it. He dreaded having to deal with new clients. His concentration at work was poor, and even routine tasks were now so much more difficult. The in-tray was slowly piling up and, for someone known for brutal efficiency, the sight of a full tray sent him into painful rumination. All sense of fun had vanished. His workmates' jokes seemed empty and meaningless. The Friday afternoon drinks were a chore, and he had stopped going to them. He did not feel connected with his family and felt guilty for feeling like this. Even his children's laughter sounded hollow. He felt that he had become a useless person, someone who had nothing to contribute and was a burden on his family and society.

Robert's agony was frozen on his countenance. The intense psychic pain was quite apparent in his expression, his voice and the way he held himself. He spoke of his dark thoughts: low hanging clouds that had turned day into night and stolen the colour from the flowers and trees. His thoughts berated him for his failings and tormented him with negative predictions of the future. He described it like being in an abyss, with no sign of a path out. Death seemed to be a welcome option to escape this misery, and the fact that he was not dying was a torment. He wished he could end it all, but he did not have the courage or the means. Even the thought of the pain his suicide would cause his family did not seem to be a strong enough reason to hang on to life.

Modern psychiatry regards this as a disorder akin to a physical disease such as diabetes. It occurs because the normal regulation of emotions has been disrupted by some aberrant process, just as abnormal glucose regulation leads to the development of diabetes. There is one big difference, however. It is easy for us to conceptualise the functioning of the body in terms of the flow of molecules and the activity of cellular function. After all, the body is but a machine. Try doing this with the mind, and we immediately become uncomfortable. This was Richard's major objection to treatment with medication. He did not want to take mind-altering drugs. I reminded him that we use drugs to change our emotions all the time. We prefer some foods that make us feel good. We drink tea to feel relaxed and alcohol for a feeling of euphoria. We do this without even thinking about brain chemistry or the mind–body problem. I saw anti-depressants in the same vein.

Richard felt differently. For him, the mind was different. I agree with him that the human mind was marvellous, because it possessed beauty, aesthetics, reason, emotion … religion, God. It was not easy to see a pill challenging all that, but it need not shake our faith in the human mind, or for that matter God. My first inclination was to dismiss Richard's anti-medication stance as being misguided. He had nevertheless nailed a problem that has preoccupied philosophers for centuries, the so-called mind–body (or mind–brain) problem.

I feel ill-equipped to carry out philosophical arguments with my patients. In fact, I consider them inappropriate, as philosophical discussions do not generally have logical conclusions. Philosophers are content with taking positions on issues and, unlike scientists, they try to muster support rather than gather evidence to knock down their pet theories. With Richard, I started with a basic premise that the mind originated from the brain. He had no difficulty with this starting point for an argument to persuade him to take an anti-depressant drug.

I needed to explain the origins of emotion to Richard – the brain as an organ of emotions just as the intestine was the organ of digestion of food and the heart the organ of circulation. This seems straightforward to us now, but has not always been the case in history. Folklore still places emotions in the heart, which we now recognise to be nothing more than a muscle required to pump the blood.

I wish to take you, the reader, on a journey of how our knowledge about the brain basis of emotions has evolved. My explanation to Richard was a lot briefer, but along similar lines.

Some of the earliest attempts to understand the origin of emotions were made by Charles Darwin.[1] As was typical of his approach, he examined the expression of emotions in animals, relying on countless sketches and photographs to show that there were some basic similarities in the way animals and humans expressed emotions. The shedding of tears when upset and baring of the teeth when angry were not unique human characteristics, but were shared by animals down the evolutionary tree. In fact, when it comes to basic emotions such as fear, anger, sadness and happiness, many features are shared, and the human expressions have vestiges in the animals. Of course, we learn a lot more about human emotions through their verbal expression, but we can accept that the lack of language is unlikely to limit the experience of the full intensity of emotion. On the contrary, we sometimes experience emotions for which we do not have the words to express. Darwin was of course interested in the survival value of emotion, and this is not hard to conceptualise. Imagine a gazelle basking in the African sun when it hears the sound of breaking twigs due to treading feet. Heaven forbid, this gazelle has no emotion – its heart does not pound, its ears do not rise in anticipation of further sounds, its leg muscles are not ready for flight and its stance is not one of complete alertness. It would certainly make a nice morsel for the lion's dinner. Its emotional arousal is fundamental to its survival. The other mechanism for survival – of the species rather than the individual – is through mating, and the procurement of a mate and the act itself are both driven by emotion. Emotions are therefore fundamental for the survival of the individual and the propagation of the species. Darwin was right in being interested in emotions.

William James,[2] the doyen of psychology in the United States, took this further in trying to explain the basis of emotions in a paper published in 1884. He argued that an exciting event, such as seeing a bear, evoked a physiological response in the body (racing heart, sweaty palms, tense muscles, dilated pupils, rapid breathing), which was perceived by the brain as the emotion of fear. In other words, the physiological response came first: we run away from the bear, then feel afraid of it. The physiological response is innate and necessary for survival. Similar ideas were proposed by Carl Lange in 1885,[3] and the theory came to be known as the James–Lange Theory of Emotion. It was extended to other emotions: we are sad because we cry and afraid because we tremble.

Understandably, many psychologists were suspicious of this theory, which gave primacy to somatic or bodily reactions rather than brain processes in the genesis of emotions. A challenge was made by Walter Cannon[4] and Philip Bard in the 1920s. They argued on the basis of a number of observations, some of which were only partially correct. Emotional behaviour in animals is preserved even when the brain is dissociated from neural inputs from the body by surgery, suggesting that the generation of emotions by the brain is not necessarily dependent on input from the body. Moreover, the physiological processes that James argued formed the basis of emotions are slow to arise, whereas emotions are often felt instantaneously. There are different types of emotions, and the physiological responses are too non-specific to account for this variety. Furthermore, if a hormone is administered to produce a physiological body response, it does not arouse the emotion generated by an emotional stimulus. The Cannon–Bard Theory[5] therefore posited that we feel the emotion first, then act on it – the basis of this feeling is of course the brain. In other words, we run from James's bear because we are afraid, and are not afraid because we run.

Cannon and Bard provided evidence to support their theory. They showed that if you removed the cortex of a cat's brain, such that it could no longer process sensory stimulation cognitively, it still generated aggressive attacks, albeit inappropriate and ill-directed ones, the so-called sham rage of the decorticate cat. They argued that the hypothalamus[6] was the brain region responsible for the generation of these responses, and in fact the higher brain regions suppressed such emotional discharges when unwelcome. However, some of the assumptions made by Cannon and Bard were incorrect. It has been shown that if the bodily organs are disconnected from the brain, the intensity of the emotion is reduced. The nature of the bodily response can at least partially distinguish the type of emotion.[7] Some hormonal manipulations of the body can induce emotion, such as the induction of panic by the infusion of cholecystokinin, a gastric hormone.

Since the data did not fully support either the James–Lange or the Cannon–Bard theories, some investigators proposed a compromise: the physiological response produced an emotional reaction, which was modified by feedback mechanisms in the brain.

The importance of the hypothalamus that Cannon and Bard had suggested was not in error. Walter Hess[8] in the 1920s implanted electrodes into the brain of a cat and showed that he could make the cat act in ways that were aggressive, fearful or curious, depending upon the region stimulated. Stimulation of one region of the hypothalamus led to alertness, increased heart rate and a propensity to attack; what he called the 'affective defence reaction'.[9] It was interesting that the full repertoire of an emotion could be produced simply by brain stimulation. Interest was thereby sparked in understanding the brain basis of emotion. The hypothalamus work had its 'logical' conclusion in the proposal of producing lesions (or destroying parts of) in the hypothalamus to control aggressive behaviour in humans,[10] a form of treatment that fortunately was abandoned, but not before several individuals had received these hypothalamotomies.

The anatomical studies set the stage for a description of the emotional regions of the brain. This was exploited brilliantly by James Papez, a neuroanatomist from the University of Minnesota, who proposed in 1937 an emotional circuit in the brain,[11] later known as the Papez Circuit. He discovered this circuit by injecting rabies virus into a cat's hippocampus and tracing its progress through the brain. The circuit involved brain regions from the hippocampus via the fornix to the mamillary bodies, the anterior thalamus and the cingulate cortex, then downstream to the hypothalamus. The front (anterior) part of the cingulate cortex is indeed a special region in this circuit. It sits like a 'collar' around the front of the corpus callosum, the fibrous bundle that connects the two cerebral hemispheres, and which we visited in chapter 2. The anatomical location and connections of the anterior cingulate cortex with other brain regions make it the ideal brain region to participate in both rational and emotional tasks, and provide a link between the two. It is the region of the brain thought to be involved in monitoring errors or conflicts between two alternatives, and helps in deciding between one of two or more choices.

Its connection with the hypothalamus suggests that it can influence the bodily response in relation to an emotion. The anterior cingulate cortex comes closest to the repository of conscious experience of the emotional state of the individual.[12] This region of the brain may be overactive or dysfunctional in some individuals with depression or anxiety disorder.

Some evidence for the role of the anterior cingulate comes from 'psychosurgery' or neurosurgery for psychiatric disorders. While psychosurgery has had a lot of bad press because of excesses of the 1950s and '60s, stereotactic surgery with focal, well-targeted lesions in the brain has been successfully used in some centres. This is not to be compared with lobotomy in which a large part of the frontal lobes was disconnected from the rest of the brain. Stereotactic psychosurgery produces small discrete lesions, and the adverse consequences are greatly reduced and in many cases altogether absent. One brain region targeted has been the anterior cingulate on both sides, called anterior cingulotomy. A group from Harvard University at Massachusetts General Hospital in Boston has had the most experience with this procedure, and they have used it to treat severe depression as well as anxiety, with good response in 30–40 per cent of cases that were resistant to all other available treatments and the illness had had a devastating effect on the individual's life. At the Neuropsychiatric Institute at the Prince of Wales Hospital in Sydney, anterior cingulotomy produced similar results in the 1970s and '80s, and the response rate was even better when the lesions were also placed in the orbito-frontal region of the brain, above the eye sockets.

If further proof was needed for the involvement of the anterior cingulate region in emotional regulation, it came from a study of deep brain stimulation to treat depression. A group of investigators from the University of Toronto, led by the neuro-psychiatrist Dr Helen Mayberg, implanted electrodes into a part of the brain close to the anterior cingulate in six patients with severe depression who had not responded to all other available treatments over a number of years.[13] The implanta-tion was done under local anaesthesia so that the patients were conscious and could report their emotional experience while still on the operating table. As soon as the current was switched on, the patients reported an immediate improvement in their emotion. The results were reproducible and did not occur with sham or placebo stimulation: 'All patients spontaneously reported acute effects including "sudden calmness or lightness," "disappearance of the void," sense of heightened awareness, increased interest, "connectedness," and sudden brightening of the room, including a description of the sharpening of visual details and intensification of colors in response to electri-cal stimulation.'[14] Four of the six patients achieved sustained improvement in their depression after six months of stimula-tion. There were metabolic changes in the brain that resembled other successful antidepressant treatments.

The Papez Circuit formed the basis for further develop-ments in the anatomy of emotion, most notably by the American neuroscientist Paul MacLean, who worked at Yale University and the National Institute of Mental Health in the United States. Not long after Papez's proposal, a paper was published by Drs Heinrich Kluver and Paul Bucy of the National Insti-tute of Neurological Disorders and Stroke in the United States. These scientists removed the temporal lobes on both sides in monkeys and noted some remarkable behavioural changes.

These monkeys, while not visually impaired, were unable to recognise even common objects (visual agnosia). They developed a strong tendency to explore their surroundings (hypermetamorphosis), and instead of using their eyes, they tended to explore objects by putting them in their mouths (oral tendencies). Their sexual behaviour changed dramatically, such that they indulged in indiscriminate sexual acts, including masturbation, and both hetero- and homosexual activity. Their emotional behaviour changed as well. They were no longer frightened of objects that would normally arouse great fear, and they freely approached humans and snakes. Their facial expressions looked more 'placid', and their vocalisations were reduced. While a full Kluver–Bucy syndrome has not been described in humans, elements of the syndrome are seen in brain-injured individuals. It was later shown by Dr Lawrence Weiskrantz,[15] a famous British psychologist known for his description of blindsight, that much of the behaviour related to Kluver–Bucy Syndrome could be produced by the removal of the amygdala on both sides. We will come back to the role of the amygdala later.

MacLean coined the term 'limbic system' in 1952. McLean had expanded the anatomical basis of emotions to include a number of other structures that formed a 'border' or limbus around the brain stem. These additional structures included the amygdala, the orbitofrontal cortex and the septal nuclei. This whole region had been labelled 'le grand lobe limbique' by Paul Broca,[16] the famous French neurologist, in 1878, but its significance for emotions was not recognised at the time. MacLean proposed the concept of the 'triune' brain whereby the brain was in reality three brains in one. The first part was the reptilian brain, which was the seat of primitive emotions

such as fear and aggression. The second was the 'old' mammalian brain, which he also referred to as the 'visceral' brain and
later the 'limbic system'. This part elaborated the primitive
emotions and was responsible for the social emotions. The
'new' mammalian brain was the latest in its evolutionary development and was responsible for higher cognition and its relationship to emotion, and was able to exert top-down control
over emotions. The three together completed the grand plan of
nature in which emotion could serve the purpose of survival
and reason could work in conjunction to elaborate or tame it
as was appropriate for the circumstances.

The concept of the emotional brain has had elaborations
and refinements in subsequent years, but the concept of the
limbic system has survived these developments. Particular focus
has been on some parts of this system: the amygdala, the insula
and the prefrontal cortex. The amygdalae (singular amygdala,
from Greek, *amygdale*, 'almond' or 'tonsil') are interesting structures lying close to the hippocampus on either side. For such
a small neural structure, it has a very complex anatomy and is
connected widely with other brain regions, especially within
the limbic system. In fact, the amygdala cannot be regarded as
one structural or functional unit, but comprises four sets of
nuclei or clumps of cells that have somewhat different functions, although they relate to each other. From being a rather
obscure structure only three decades ago, it has now entered
lay parlance as the seat of fear. Some classic work by the New
York University neuroscientist Joseph LeDoux showed that
amygdala is central to the acquisition of fear conditioning in
the rat.[17] In the conditioning experiment, the rat is exposed
to an emotionally neutral stimulus such as a tone – called the

conditioned stimulus or CS – which is paired with an unconditioned stimulus (US) such as an electric shock. The brain is
already tuned to respond to an electric shock with fear. When
the pairing is repeated a few times, the CS also begins to elicit
the same behavioural response as the US. The tone now makes
the rat become alert, in a defensive posture with increased heart
rate, raised blood pressure and the pumping of noradrenalin
in the system. LeDoux and colleagues showed that the amygdala was essential for conditioning to occur. The conditioning
experiment is akin to the sound of the breaking twig alerting
the gazelle to the presence of a predator. Of course, in situations such as this, the brain must work quickly for the flight
response to be fast enough for survival. The sensory information from the ears, after passing through the relay station in the
thalamus, reaches the amygdala both directly and indirectly via
the cerebral cortex. LeDoux has referred to these as the 'low'
road (the direct thalamo-amygdala route) and the 'high' road
(the thalamo-cortico-amygdala route). The lower information
highway favours the quick response, but does not permit cognitive processing of the information – something that might save
the life of the gazelle. The high road might decide that this is a
false alarm after processing this and other information coming
through the various sensory organs.

The precise experiments that can be conducted in laboratory animals are not possible in humans, but neuroimaging
technology now permits similar questions to be addressed in
humans. It has been shown in functional MRI studies that the
processing of emotional stimuli such as faces with emotional
expressions, especially those manifesting fear, activate the amygdala. A similar activation is not seen with happy faces. Scott

Rauch and colleagues at the Massachusetts General Hospital in Boston conducted studies to determine the brain response when fearful stimuli were shown to individuals, and demonstrated that activation of the amygdala was an integral feature of the brain's response.[18] Individuals in whom the amygdala has been damaged have difficulty in detecting emotion in other people's faces. If the amygdala is damaged on both sides, the individual has difficulty learning fear, as in the classical conditioning experiments. This was shown elegantly by Bechara and colleagues, who examined three individuals, the first with damage to both amygdala, the second with damage to both hippocampi, and the third in whom both structures were damaged.[19] The individuals with amygdala damage were unable to acquire fear conditioning – the unconditioned stimulus was a loud tone, which caused a startle-like response, and the conditioning stimulus was the colour blue – but they were able to remember which colour was paired with which stimulus. The individual with hippocampal damage acquired the conditioning but was unable to remember the facts.

Such a role for the amygdala has clinical and real-life significance. It is possible that it is the amygdala that alerts the brain to the possibility of a snake when it 'sees' a rope on the jungle path in the twilight. The amygdala responds to the shadows in the dark on a lonely road. Much of this response is adaptive, and can be suitably contained by the rational part of the brain. This is not the case in phobic individuals in whom an otherwise harmless stimulus evokes such panic that a crisis is signalled. The mere sight of a spider, or being caught in a lift, or having to board a flight can be such stimuli in phobic individuals. For the anorexic young woman, the sight of food can produce an activation of the amygdala, evoking a fear response that results in avoidance of food.

The amygdala is also responsible for enhancing emotion-laden memories. It is a common observation that we have clear memories of past events that had a strong emotional impact on us: the first kiss, the place of proposal for marriage, the time when you heard of a loved one's death – all are indelibly imprinted in the memory stores. Most people will be able to answer the question: where were you when the news of Princess Diana's (or JFK's) death broke? These are events unlike any other as they produce a strong emotional arousal, and it has repeatedly been shown that arousal facilitates memory. The amygdala plays a critical role in this. Unfortunately, it over-shoots the mark in certain circumstances. The memory of a terrible accident is something that we would rather erase from our minds, but the amygdala makes sure that it is deeply ingrained, and some individuals relive it with the re-experience of the arousal that it was originally associated with – the situation of post-traumatic stress disorder. Many a war veteran will attest to the distressing and overwhelming nature of such memories, which persist without serving any purpose in the long term. Since arousal is an integral part of the laying down of such memories, it has been suggested that drugs that reduce arousal – such as the anti-adrenergic drug propranolol – might help in reducing the impact of traumatic events if given soon after the event, for example to rape victims or road accident victims in the Emergency Room.

Another interesting part of the emotional brain is the insula[20] (from Latin, meaning 'island') – a part of the cerebral cortex that lies between the temporal, frontal and parietal lobes and in fact is covered by portions of these lobes called the 'opercula' (or 'lids'). Its anatomical position and its extensive connections with the thalamus as well as the amygdala result in input of various sensory modalities – pain, temperature, touch, hearing, smell, taste, state of bodily organs, musculoskeletal system, oxygen status – as well as emotional state. It has therefore been suggested that the insula may represent the subjective emotional experience[21] by monitoring the bodily state that accompanies such emotion. Desires such as food or drug craving activate the insula, and in drug users, environmental cues for drug taking are sufficient to activate this region. It was shown in one study that individuals who meditate have a thicker insula on the right,[22] which may explain their ability to better monitor their bodily states and keep their emotions on an even keel. It is perhaps too simplistic to localise the concept of the 'self' in any brain region, but if any region comes close to the embodiment of this concept, it is the insula, and it may well be the basis of the 'gut feeling' that we so often depend upon in our lives. Activity in the insula was abnormal in Anna, the young lady with anorexia we met in chapter 5.

The third brain region that deserves special mention is the prefrontal cortex, the part of the brain involved in highest mental functions and which interacts closely with emotions. The prefrontal cortex is of course a large region and comprises many subregions, each with some degree of specialisation. We have already talked about the prefrontal cortex in relation to Stephen's problems in chapter 6. Antonio Damasio and his colleagues from the University of Iowa placed a special emphasis on the role of the ventromedial prefrontal cortex that sits close to the midline. It is closely connected to the amygdala and exercises some degree of control over it. It is responsible for the extinction of the emotional conditioning achieved by the amygdala. While the memory of past events is still present, the prefrontal cortex helps reduce the emotional valence attached to the memory. This region of the cortex is also the basis for the processing of 'somatic markers', according to Damasio. These markers tag the physiological state of the body to certain emotional states, thereby providing a somatic code for emotions. This helps the individual to navigate through situations of uncertainty and make decisions on the basis of 'gut feeling', so to speak. Damasio argued in his book *Descartes' Error* that decision-making, especially in situations of uncertainty, is highly influenced by the emotional state of the individual, and somatic markers are particularly important for this.

This was demonstrated in Elliott,[23] a man in his thirties who developed a brain tumour close to the midline just above his eyes, which affected both frontal lobes. The tumour had to be removed and, along with it, brain tissue from both frontal lobes. The University of Iowa researchers tested Elliott at some length in the subsequent months. Surprisingly, he performed well on most formal neuropsychological tests. His intelligence quotient (IQ) was placed in the superior range, and he performed well on tasks of short-term memory, past memory, new learning, language function, arithmetic ability, ability to focus attention and retain information on-line (working memory) and some tests of frontal lobe function. In fact, he could perform the Wisconsin Card Sort test quite well. In this test, a person is asked to categorise a pack of cards according to one of three principles (colour, shape or number), and the examiner changes the categorising principle without warning, and the testee has to quickly realise the shift in the strategy according to the new principle. It tests a person's ability to sort into categories and shift the mental set flexibly, something that Elliott was able to do. He was also able to make estimates in mental manipulations and make estimates based on incomplete knowledge. Yet his social and personal functioning was devastatingly affected. He managed his time at work poorly, and moved from one activity to another without completing the previous one and without appreciating the consequences of this behaviour. He would sometimes spend many hours deliberating over an inconsequential matter, and was unable to prioritise. He began to collect seemingly useless items. He started new business ventures without planning and teamed up with disreputable individuals against whom he had been forewarned, subsequently losing all his savings.

Damasio used cases like Elliott's to argue for the role of emotion in decision-making. The effect of the tumour on Elliott meant he had lost the passion that goes with many of life's travails. He no longer showed impatience or frustration when his work was thwarted, or eagerness or enthusiasm when an event demanded immediate action. He was little moved by gory accidents, burning houses or earthquakes! The region of the brain that informed his decision-making with strong emotion had been damaged, and his decisions were now bereft of the guidance of emotions that he had depended upon throughout his life.

While his IQ had been mostly unaffected, he had lost much of his emotional intelligence (EI). The concept of emotional intelligence has been around since the time of Charles Darwin, but it was resurrected more recently by Peter Salovey and John

'Jack' Mayer,[24] and popularised by Daniel Goleman.[25] Elliott had a high IQ but a low EQ (emotional quotient), making him good at test performance but a failure in real life. In such individuals, self-awareness and self-expression are affected, and these individuals are not able to navigate effectively in social situations. Their judgment in social and interpersonal situations is affected, resulting in an inability to effectively solve problems and make decisions in such situations. A number of related concepts have been talked about. The term 'alexithymia' (from Greek, literally 'without words for emotions') was introduced by the psychotherapist Peter Sifneos to describe individuals who had difficulty in understanding and expressing their emotions. These individuals were thought to make poor subjects for psychotherapy and tended to develop somatic disorders, such as chronic pain. Other terms such as 'psychological mindedness', 'empathy', 'practical intelligence' and 'successful intelligence' overlap with the concept of EI. The term 'theory of mind' was introduced to denote an individual's ability to attribute beliefs, intents or desires to oneself and others, and to understand that others have beliefs, desires and intentions that are different from one's own.[26] This again has much to do with EI.

Why have I not mentioned depression in my discussion of the anatomy of emotions? Is depression really a fundamental emotion? Does it have a purpose in nature? Why do some individuals become trapped in it? And, of course, how can a pill working on a brain chemical get the person out of such a state?

Depression is so prevalent in society and throughout

culture and history that it must serve a useful function in human evolution. A number of social biologists have argued that depression as an emotion must have an adaptive function, although depression severe enough to present as a clinical syndrome is most certainly maladaptive. In a hierarchical society such as that of some primates, the depressive stance of submissiveness would be an appropriate response to loss of social status to the alpha male.[27] The slowing down of the body in depression could be a way of conserving energy to recover from the struggle for domination that preceded it. The struggle, however, may not have been for domination but for survival in an adversity. The social response of caring and compassion that depression usually generates is arguably adaptive for the social grouping and increases the networked cohesion of the group. An individual may, in fact, use it to his advantage by manipulating the feelings of others or use the time to reflect on new ways of behaving. Drs Matthew Kessler of the University of California at Los Angeles and Randolph Nesse of the University of Michigan at Ann Arbor[28] argued that different symptoms of depression may have different adaptive functions. According to this theory, low mood is aversive and, since it often follows a loss, it prevents actions that might bring about future losses. Individuals may avoid certain actions or situations for fear of a loss that would induce low mood, thereby pre-empting the loss. Crying is a powerful social signal that elicits help and strengthens a social network. Self-reproach signals culpability to others and may avoid the loss of social bonds. Fatigue may help conserve energy in situations in which activity is unlikely to have a positive pay-off. Pessimism one sees as part of depression prevents future action that has already proven to be futile. Loss of appetite would reduce foraging in uncertain situations, thereby preserving the individual, and loss of sleep might protect against predators and other threats. This is of course all speculative, and there are many counterpoints to each of the arguments raised. What cannot be doubted is that the brain has a neural system that underlies depression.

The precise neural basis of depression is not understood, but neuroscientists have again looked to the limbic system in order to understand depression. I have already mentioned some of the important structures above. The network of brain structures has had to be extended to account for many of the clinical features of depression.[29] Many clinicians are struck by the fact that depression is a common complication in disorders that affect the basal ganglia[30] (or basal nuclei): large clumps of neurons that sit in the middle of the brain and are connected to the cerebral cortex and the thalamus, forming what are known as cortico-subcortical circuits. It has been known for some time that strokes affecting the basal ganglia may result in the development of depression. Huntington's disease is a neuro-degenerative disease that preferentially affects the neurons in the basal ganglia initially. The basal ganglia have complex structures with multiple functions, and their primary role has in the past been considered to be related to movement. They are relative newcomers in the field of emotion and thinking, but have now firmly established their place, and might be the key to the understanding of the effects of certain drugs. The volumes of the caudate nuclei – key parts of the basal ganglia – are smaller in patients with severe depression. It must be hurriedly mentioned that the frontal cortex, the basal ganglia and the thalamus from part of a network or circuit – six such circuits were described by Alexander and colleagues in one of the most cited papers in neuroscience.[31]

The other region of much interest in depression is the prefrontal cortex, the large brain area that I have already discussed above. All three major parts of the prefrontal cortex – the dorsolateral region that sits on the side, the anterior cingulate region that sits in the middle and the orbitofrontal region that sits at the bottom, just above the eye sockets – have been implicated in depression. The more consistent findings have been reduced activity in the dorsolateral and anterior cingulate regions, although some studies have shown increased activity in the cingulate region. Studies of the orbitofrontal region tend to show increased activity in this region. These abnormalities might explain why depressed individuals are poorly motivated to begin new tasks or maintain something that they have already started, and why their attention cannot be sustained for long enough for them to work effectively. This disturbance may be so severe in some cases that they may be diagnosed as suffering from dementia, especially if they are older. In most cases, when asked to perform a task that uses this brain region, they are able to temporarily overcome the difficulty and raise the activity level in the prefrontal brain regions.[32] More importantly, it has been shown that the treatment of depression results in the establishment of normal levels of prefrontal activation, and it does not seem to matter which form of treatment is being used: drug treatment or cognitive behaviour therapy or brain stimulation, all achieve the same goal.

I think that the neuronal networks or circuits that underpin the emotional state were dysfunctional in Richard's brain. I could not tell him where exactly the abnormality was or the precise nature of that abnormality. It was possible that his prefrontal cortex was 'stuck' in a mode of reduced function and was unable to modulate his emotion out of its depressed state. It could well be that the basal ganglia were at fault, which in turn would affect the function in the thalamus and thereby the prefrontal cortex through the feedback loop.

I tried to explain it to him thus: 'Imagine that the brain networks that are the basis of your emotional state normally have a certain level of function in them, producing a "neural state" that corresponds to your usual "mental state". It is not the same in everybody, as all of us do not feel the same – or so I believe. Moreover, we do not feel the same all the time. I have some fluctuations in my mood through the day: I feel lousy leaving my bed and am full of enthusiasm and positive emotions in the early afternoon. This may be due to some rhythms in the neural states. The neural state also goes through some turbulence. I hear bad news – my grant application was unsuccessful – and my neural state changes to put me in a blue mood. However, this is still reactive to the environment: the warm smile of my daughter quickly puts the grant failure behind me and lightens up my being. The brain states can be said to be plastic: they move with the times, and respond to the environment in a flexible sort of way. However, there is a bias in these states to revert to their "natural" state – whatever is natural for that individual.'

I regard depression as the persistence of an abnormal neural state: the brain is stuck in the wrong gear and has temporarily lost the ability to revert to neutral. This abnormal state can to some extent be captured by a positron emission scan, which measures the metabolic activity in different brain regions. The reduced activity in the prefrontal cortex is one component of such a neural state. Of course this is still a crude measure given the complexity of the underlying biology. A neural state is nothing but the level of information processing in a certain network of neurons, and in this case the network that underlies depressed mood. The network is quite complex, and we understand it only superficially. Our attempts to deal with the abnormal function are therefore crude relative to the sophistication of the neuronal connections.

But where does a drug like Prozac (fluoxetine) fit in the scheme of things? Let us call it gear oil to loosen the system, or a stirrer to set things in motion once again. The neural system in a depressive state needs a nudge or a push to start moving again, and Prozac provides that momentum. Now, why an 'antidepressant' like Prozac and not some other drug? As a matter of fact, Prozac is not unique in having this property. This is where brain chemistry comes into play.

Many a depressed patient has been told by a doctor that their brain is low in serotonin[33] and that they need to take a drug that brings up the level of this chemical. This should be regarded as a metaphor rather than a statement of fact. For one, the evidence is not strong that serotonin levels are indeed low in the brains of depressed individuals. Measuring brain levels of a chemical in a living human brain is indeed a major challenge. There are some imaging techniques available, but they tell us about the levels of receptors for a particular chemical rather than the chemical itself. Scientists have tried to overcome the difficulty by measuring the metabolites of serotonin in the cerebrospinal fluid, which is an indicator of how much serotonin is being produced by the brain.

When serotonin is secreted by a nerve ending, most of it is taken up by the secreting cell itself, and only a small fraction is broken down. An important breakdown substance is 5HIAA (5-hydroxy indole acetic acid), which can be measured. The story becomes complicated again because this metabolite is in small quantities in the spinal fluid and its level may be influenced by extraneous factors such as time of day, whether or not the person has been sleeping well and their diet. Not surprisingly, the results in depressed individuals have been far from consistent, and this line of investigation has been largely abandoned. The only exception is suicide – the spinal fluid of individuals who have recently attempted suicide have shown lower levels of the metabolite, but suicide should not be equated with depression as many people who attempt suicide do not have a depressive illness, and the lower levels may be a consequence rather than a cause of the suicide.

When direct measurement proved frustrating, scientists resorted to another method of determining the role of lower levels of serotonin. Serotonin is manufactured by the body from the dietary amino acid tryptophan. Amino acids are the building blocks of proteins, and some amino acids are regarded as essential as they cannot be synthesised by the human body and must be ingested. Fortunately, a number of dietary substances are rich in tryptophan, and these include milk, chocolate, bananas, poultry, fish, red meat, sesame, chickpeas, sunflower seeds and peanuts. In addition to building proteins, tryptophan in the body is metabolised to serotonin and melatonin. It is interesting that tryptophan has been promoted as a sleep-inducing agent in the lay press, although the evidence for this is weak. Since serotonin is promoted as a calming neurotransmitter, and melatonin is a sleep-inducing hormone produced by the pineal gland in response to darkness, a precursor of these two substances is justifiably of interest as a sleep-inducing drug. It has been available in health stores for this purpose for many years. In 1989 tryptophan was linked to a large outbreak of an autoimmune illness called eosinophilia-myalgia syndrome, which affected 1500 individuals and led to 37 deaths. In 1991 tryptophan was banned by the Federal Drugs Administration in the United States, followed by other countries, even though the adverse effect was linked to one batch of tryptophan from a Japanese manufacturer. Tryptophan is still available over the counter in many countries, but its popularity with the medical profession has waned as consequence of the scare. The popular press continues to promote it. Some urban myths abound, one of which is the somnolent effects of a turkey dinner on Thanksgiving. The so-called turkey coma is due to a hefty dose of tryptophan. In one episode of *Seinfeld*, Jerry and George caused Jerry's girlfriend to fall asleep with turkey and boxed wine so that they could play with her toy collection. In *Reno 911*, another American TV series, tryptophan is claimed to be as dangerous as alcohol for driving. Blaming turkey is peculiar as it has no more tryptophan than poultry in general, and is comparable to red meat and fish. It is most likely the carbohydrate in the meal that produces the drowsiness.[34]

Neuroscientists were interested in the effects of reducing serotonin in the brain to see if it induced depression. It was shown in the mid-1970s that giving a tryptophan-free diet can lead to a rapid depletion of brain tryptophan and serotonin. The effect of this in healthy individuals and depressed patients has now been tested in a large number of studies.[35] In healthy individuals, the lowering of tryptophan by dietary means does not induce depression, nor does it do so in depressed patients who have recovered and are no longer on drug treatment. In patients who are well but are still being maintained on drugs, this drug challenge leads to a relapse of their depression. These studies suggest that we cannot equate low serotonin with depression *per se*, but the fact that those on treatment relapse supports the view that the drugs do need high levels of serotonin for their action. There are some individuals – those with a family history of depression or some other marker of genetic vulnerability to depression – who do show some lowering of mood with tryptophan depletion. Serotonin depletion must therefore work in a brain that is vulnerable to becoming depressed because of its genetic make-up.

This is all understandable! Serotonin is important, but it is only part of the story. The first antidepressant drug, iproniazid, was discovered by serendipity as it was manufactured for the treatment of tuberculosis. When it was shown to help depression, its mechanism of action came under scrutiny, and the first class of antidepressants – the monoamine oxidase inhibitors (MAOIs) – was established. These drugs worked on the enzyme MAO, which is responsible for breaking down serotonin and norepinephrine in the brain, leading to higher levels of both these neurotransmitters. The chemical hypothesis of depression was born by reverse logic: if drugs that increased the levels of these chemicals in the brain led to improvement of depression, then depression must be because of a deficiency of these chemicals. This was an appealing hypothesis. It was supported by the evidence from the next class of antidepressants – the tricyclics – which were shown to block the uptake of serotonin and norepinephrine by the releasing neuron, thereby increasing their availability at the nerve terminal where its action is located. Further advances in antidepressant treatment have mostly focused on this property – reuptake inhibition for serotonin or norepinephrine – and these newer drugs have been shown to be effective, albeit no more than the older drugs, but with fewer side effects. It was in an attempt to achieve drugs with less side effects that the more selective drugs were manufactured; the modern phase of drug development beginning in 1987 with the approval of Prozac (or fluoxetine), a serotonin-specific reuptake inhibitor (SSRI).

A complicating factor in this story is that the antidepressant effect is not restricted to manipulation of serotonin levels. The same can be achieved in many patients by manipulating the levels of norepinephrine and, to a lesser extent, dopamine. Some of the tricyclic antidepressants work largely, if not exclusively, on norepinephrine reuptake, and in the mid-1990s the drug reboxetine (Edronax) was introduced as an antidepressant that works exclusively on norepinephrine. The results produced by tryptophan depletion are also produced by the acute depletion of phenylalanine and tyrosine, amino acids necessary for the synthesis of norepinephrine and dopamine. How does one reconcile this with the serotonin hypothesis of depression? Are there two or more kinds of depression, based on their neurochemistry? Is it horses for courses when choosing a drug for a depressed patient? The evidence does not clearly point to this kind of a distinction between patients. Now, what about a drug that increases reuptake of serotonin – a pharmacological effect opposite to that of SSRI drugs? Would it worsen depression? One such drug is available in Europe – tianeptine (Stablon,[36]

Coaxil, Tatinol) – and, surprisingly, it is an effective antidepressant. It is a wounding blow to a simple chemical hypothesis.

Let's throw in another complicating factor: the time course of antidepressant action. One of my first warnings to Richard was not to expect an immediate response to the medication. I generally tell my patients: 'The drug will initially make you feel worse – because of the side effects – before it starts making you better ever so gradually.' The reuptake block in the brain occurs within minutes to hours, but the antidepressant effect typically takes weeks. A likely explanation is that the primary drug effect starts a cascade of other effects that eventually result in the relief of depression. Some of the focus has been on molecules that come into action when a neurotransmitter such as serotonin or norepinephrine acts on a receptor – the so-called second and third messengers in a chain of molecules. Investigation of these has led to some wonderful insights but without explaining the antidepressant effect satisfactorily. The other result of excess serotonin in the synapse[37] (the point of coming together of one nerve cell with another) is that receptors on the receiving neuron are modified so that they become less responsive (are 'down-regulated') – the net result being that the information transmission is reduced. Many neuro-scientists have argued that this is the long-term end-point that we wish to reach with anti-depressants, and accounts for the delay of onset of their action. Some investigators have argued that there is no delay in the onset of action of the drugs,[38] but the early changes are subtle and not clinically apparent, and the effect becomes appreciable only after a delay because it has to cross the 'clinical' threshold. Even they will accept that it is a gradual process that does not reach its peak until some weeks have elapsed.

This brings us to a quotation from Arvid Carlsson's Nobel lecture:[39] 'However, it must be recognized that the brain is not a chemical factory but an extremely complicated survival machine. In order to bring all the forthcoming biochemical observations into a meaningful framework it will prove meaningful to emphasize more strongly aspects of neurocircuits and connectivity and to do so both at the microscopic and macroscopic level.'[40]

Chemicals are merely messengers in the overall complexity of neuronal circuits, and it is the disturbance in the circuit itself that is likely to be the immediate antecedent of the mental state. Serotonin, norepinephrine and dopamine have a particular distribution in the brain that reflects their diverse effects. These chemicals originate in the brain stem in small clumps of specialised nerve cells and send fibres that connect with various brain regions, including the limbic system, the basal ganglia and the cortex. They may be regarded as the brain's watering systems, which set the tone of activity in various regions.

They also have a role in brain development and its plasticity. If antidepressants are given to animals soon after birth, they produce some permanent changes in brain development, leading to lasting behavioural disturbances in adulthood. Antidepressants in adult life may produce some plastic brain changes. It has been shown that these drugs promote the formation of new nerve cells in some brain regions, in particular the hippocampus, and also cause an increase in connections of existing cells. The formation of new cells (neurogenesis) by antidepressants has caused a great deal of excitement in neuroscience. It used to be believed that the adult brain did not form new cells, but this dogma has now definitely been proven incorrect. It would seem that a depressed brain is attempting to repair or reset its network by modifying old cells and forming new ones, and the drugs assist in the process. How they do this is unknown, but new insights are gradually emerging. One possibility is that antidepressants activate some chemicals that are neurotrophins – they modify brain connections both in the developing and adult brains. One such factor that has received attention is the brain-derived neurotrophic factor (BDNF), activity of which is increased in the hippocampus and cortex by antidepressant drugs.[41]

The brain is a living active organism that is changing constantly. It used to be thought that most brain regions were immutable – once developed, they changed very little except for loss that occurred with ageing. In the last 20 years, we have come to realise that the brain is constantly responding to environmental stimuli and rewiring itself. The plasticity of brain circuits can extend to such activities as meditation, emotional experiences and behaviour therapy. Drugs must be seen in this context as aids in the process of plasticity. It is quite possible that electroconvulsive therapy (ECT, the so-called shock therapy) produces its effects through similar mechanisms.

Following some of my explanations, Richard was more open to considering medication for his treatment, but his mind still harboured some doubts. He was willing to accept that the mechanism of action of these drugs is probably more complex than a simple enhancement of serotonin. He was worried about neurogenesis and the possible formation of new synapses (synaptogenesis). Questions were welling up in his mind: if these drugs are helping form new nerve cells and their connections, how can we be certain that these will indeed be beneficial? Could they not be harmful – after all, more cannot necessarily be better? Could these harmful effects, if they do occur, be permanent?

He was posing questions to which I did not have good answers. I had to agree with him that more neurogenesis and synaptogenesis could not be considered inherently beneficial. After all, at the age of four years, we have twice as many neurons as we do when we are adults, yet the adult brain functions much more effectively. I had to appeal to the goodness of Mother Nature. I agreed that more neurons did not equate with better function. The newly formed neurons must be integrated within neuronal circuits so that the flow of information is smooth and efficient. In computer terms, it could be understood as signal-to-noise ratio, or SNR. Any new developments should improve the SNR of the emotional system. We must finally rely on the brain's capacity to normalise itself, with the drug merely aiding the process.

But how do we know that the brain is repairing itself? Is it not abnormal in its function such that it cannot maintain the normal mood state? Let us take an event that makes you sad. Suppose your dog is run over by a car. You feel sad, your appetite goes and you lose the motivation to go to work that day. Your brain can be said to have gone into a depressed mode. When you get up the next day, you are not as depressed, and you try to be philosophical about it. It was an accident – it was not something that you could have prevented – life goes on – you have to be strong for your kids, who are devastated by the loss. Various thoughts go through your mind. You go to work, and soon become absorbed in the routine of the day. You even think of getting another dog. And, in a few days time, the negative emotion that tinged your memory of your dog becomes less painful. Your brain has reset itself back to normal. Perhaps some factors in the environment have helped the process. The day off, the ritual of burying the dog, the support of your family, and the few tears that you shed might all have helped the brain to reset itself, but its capacity is well demonstrated. You could even say that the brain is biased toward resetting itself to its routine state.

Would Richard's brain, troubled as it was, also reset itself with time? Previous experience is that this is quite likely, but it may take many months if no help is offered. I did not advocate this path to Richard – it would entail a great deal of suffering, and there is a possibility that being in this state is not good for the brain. A prolonged state of depression could in fact damage the brain for a number of reasons. The longer the brain is in a particular state, the more difficult it could become to completely reverse that state. Being in the state of depression has other consequences as well. Since the body is in a state of stress, it is pumping out some hormones. The most noteworthy is cortisol, a hormone produced by the adrenal glands in response to another hormone pumped out by the pituitary gland in the brain. Cortisol is the prototypical stress hormone – it prepares the body for stress such as fever, surgery, extreme exertion or action in battle. There is good evidence that high levels of cortisol, when they persist for too long, may damage the brain. One region that is most vulnerable to this damage is the hippocampus, so important for memory. It was therefore in Richard's long-term interest to treat his depression as soon as possible.

I had persuaded Richard that he needed treatment fairly urgently, but how did I know which one was better for him: drug treatment or cognitive behaviour therapy (CBT)? And, if a drug, which one?

The answer to these questions was based on the results of treatment studies that have been conducted around the world, and from my own experience of hundreds of patients I had treated in the past. Of course, clinical experience is not always objective, and one can reinforce one's biases by paying attention to selective information. There are some ground rules that most clinicians follow – the nature of his depression suggested to me that drug treatment should be the primary treatment modality. As his condition improved, I would engage him in CBT while maintaining his drug treatment. Drug treatment and CBT are not exclusive of each other, and both can work synergistically.

Richard and his wife wanted to know whether they had to make changes to their lives. Their reasoning was simple: 'After all, if I am depressed, there must be something wrong with my life or how I face it!' It brings us back to the question: how much of this problem was due to Richard's vulnerability to depression, and how much was caused by an environmental stress? It is best to regard the brain and the environment as an interacting dyad. You can have a brain very prone to becoming depressed, but could live such a glorious life that a situation severe enough to cause depression never arises. On the other hand, a very robust neural system – a Nelson Mandela – can overcome the most extreme of stresses and still come out victorious. Most of us lie somewhere in between these two extremes.

It seemed to me that Richard was more towards the vulnerable end: not much appeared to have happened to stress him, yet he found himself in this predicament. His next question was the obvious one: why me? He had seen his friends go through the most horrific of life's difficulties, and it was water off the duck's back to them.

The answer most definitely lay, at least partly, in his genes. From studies in twins, it would appear that genes account for at least a third of the risk for depression.[42] Some interesting data emerged from a study in New Zealand, the Dunedin Birth Cohort. The investigators of this study found that variation on one gene had a major influence on whether an individual developed depression in response to a stressful live event.[43] This gene codes for the serotonin transporter, the protein that determines how much serotonin is taken back into the nerve cell that secretes it at the synapse. The gene comes in two forms: short (S) or long (L), giving the combinations SS, SL or LL. Having the S form of the gene – called allele in technical terms – makes the protein less efficient. The study found that the occurrence of depression or suicide attempts after a stressful event was significantly greater in those with the SS or the SL genes, but not in the LL carriers. The S allele did not itself cause depression – it made the brain respond to stress with less resilience. This finding was replicated by many other groups around the world, including my colleagues at the University of New South Wales, led by Professor Kay Wilhelm, who has been following a group of teachers for nearly three decades through the travails and tribulations of their lives. It has been shown in mice as well – those with the S version had a greater response to stress as measured by the level of cortisol in the blood. In another interesting study, it was shown that those with SS or SL alleles activated their amygdala to a greater extent than the LL when exposed to fearful stimuli. This is just one example of how our genetic make-up can make us more or less vulnerable. The interesting point is that the genes interact with the environment, and both must be present for the effect to occur.

Could Richard get some genetic testing done to see whether he was SS or SL? Indeed, shouldn't we all get this testing done so that we are aware of our risk? I am afraid the answer is not that simple. While it is possible to test a person for S and L alleles, and the cost is not prohibitive, I do not think it would help a great deal. At this stage, we cannot predict how many people with the vulnerability gene will develop depression and under what circumstances. No life can be totally free of stress – even being suspended in a bubble, with your nutritional needs being adequately met, might be quite stressful. Stress for one person may be a walk through the park for another, and what is stressful at one phase of life may be quite welcome at another. There may be some ways in which we can inoculate ourselves against stress. Exposure to stress in small doses, which we overcome effectively, increases our ability to tolerate stress in the future. We could also increase our resilience through meditation or positive mentalising or religion or a number of other ways. Some investigators are developing a preventative psychiatry, teaching how to deal with crises early so that long-term damage is obviated. It can be argued that those of us who are SS should work harder at this, but the rules apply to all of us. Let us wait for more information before we rush to get ourselves genetically tested. We will also need some reassurance that our insurance companies will not take

advantage of this information and raise the premiums for the
SSs and SLs in society.

I persuaded Richard that genetic testing was not in his best
interest. He would need to reduce his stress levels and work on
his resilience no matter what – but he must wait until he has
recovered from the current depression.

Richard did decide to take medication. He started on a small
dose, which was increased to a 'therapeutic' dose within two
weeks. When I saw him six weeks later he was feeling much
less depressed. There was more spirit in his speech. He walked
more briskly, and his face had regained some of its lost animus.
The tone of his voice showed more variability. He felt that
the darkness was beginning to lift. He now decided to go for
CBT and continue the medication. I saw him regularly for
about six months, and he had weekly sessions with a clinical
psychologist for 12 weeks. At the end of this period, he had
returned to work and the depression had settled completely.
He had made changes to his work routine to reduce the level
of stress. He had been reading the teachings of the Dalai Lama
and was confident of achieving equanimity in his life. When I
finally referred him back to his family doctor, my task appeared
to be over. His parting shot: 'Dr Sachdev, I had to work on
my depression – but the medication did help! I cannot decide
which was more important.'

8

A chesty problem

*The most crippling obsessions create absurd, embarrassing, or
frightening thoughts that repeat in the mind in an endless loop ...
Perhaps the most painful aspect is the insight my patients have
about the absurdity and the wastefulness of the crazy thoughts that
consume their lives.*

Dr Judith Rapoport, *The Boy Who Couldn't Stop Washing*[1]

We place a huge premium on the flexibility of our thinking.
We are impressed by individuals who are 'quick' of mind,
the Robyn Williamses of this world. They can respond to a
situation with speed and alacrity – and often creativity – and
do not seem to be paralysed by doubt and indecision. They
are able to weigh up conflicting information without endless
rounds of deliberation. They do not unnecessarily ponder over
the may-be's or the what-if's. The flow of thought in such
minds is swift and unidirectional, not unlike a stream bubbling
and rushing down the mountains, which can change direction
at the hint of a thwarting stone and create marvellous pools
in the most insignificant crevices. There is a certain freshness
about such minds that makes us envious.

This flexibility of the mind is an innate property of the
brain. The balance between the brain regions involved in the

process of weighing options, then choosing one of them to conclude the decision-making process, must be fine and delicate, and is achieved more easily by some individuals than others. Philip was not such a person. At 25 years of age, he could look back to many years when his mind had been fettered by doubt and indecision. As a child he remembered that he could move along with the flow. His mother, Mrs Headingly, described him as a serious child, but one who did enjoy the usual pleasures of childhood. These were comforting memories for a mother: how he would play in the park with children from the neighbourhood, the wild manner in which he rode his bicycle, the mess his clothes would be in when he returned from school and the spontaneous laughter and cheekiness that can be so endearing at that age. She was that rare mother who was wistful of the disorganised little child Philip once was. Even at the early age of seven or eight years, there were signs of something developing inside his mind that would make these childhood foibles just joyful memories.

It started with little rituals that seemed innocent and even amusing. Philip's mother liked to put him to bed, but from the age of about eight, Philip insisted that she come into his room only when he had finished undressing. This seemed like an innocent request of a young boy and the assertion of his growing independence. When this became increasingly prolonged, it began to frustrate his mother. Philip had developed a special 'way' of changing into his nightclothes and arranging his bed sheets. Each article of clothing when removed had to be folded neatly and placed in his cupboard. His pants were always folded first, followed by the jumper and the shirt. He had been instructed by his mother that his underclothes were to be placed in the laundry chute every night. Even these were folded, and Philip insisted that he would walk these to the laundry rather than use the convenience of the chute. Mrs Headingly thought this odd but did not make an issue of it. What did frustrate her was the increasing amount of time Philip was taking to get ready for bed.

Mrs Headingly took pride in her little boy who was becoming increasingly responsible as he was growing up. His school bag was always in order in the mornings, and his school uniform was neatly folded by his bed. She could afford to indulge his slowness at bedtime, although in her frustration she did call out and sometimes knock on his door to hurry him up. There was no sense that a problem was building up ever so slowly. Philip's work at school was exemplary. His teacher could depend upon him to always complete his homework, to keep his notebooks tidy, and to turn up for all the extracurricular activities. He was becoming more serious, however. He did not participate in the silliness and histrionic behaviour of the other boys in the class. His 'maturity' appeared to be beyond his years.

Concern was first raised by his teacher when he was 10 years old. His work was tidy and accurate, but there were days when only half of it had been completed. He was noted to check his work again and again, making certain that no word had been misspelled and the calculations were all correct. He did not complain about it, but when the teacher prompted him to hurry up in class, he tended to become tense and one day burst into tears. A parent–teacher interview followed, but neither party had recognised the core problem. Philip's father had been absent from home a great deal in relation to his work – perhaps Philip was missing his father. The teacher reduced his homework, and his father decided to spend more time with him. His work improved, and his parents declared victory. No professional consultation resulted.

Philip remembered his final years at school as having been happy. He remained the serious but nice kid who worked hard and had impeccable manners. There was no teenage rebellion or late-night parties. He was growing into a handsome young man, with his father's looks and physique. His focus had shifted from his school work to his appearance. His father bought him weights for his sixteenth birthday, and he began to spend more than an hour on weight-training every day. The results initially pleased his parents, but when he began training early in the morning, and was often late for school, they were worried. They initially tried to convince themselves that this was a teen-age concern with appearance that would wane as he matured. Training began to take over much of the time at home. The garage, where the weights were kept, had become a gym. He would disappear into it for hours at weekends. A family meet-ing followed at which his parents demanded that he stick to a strict routine in relation to his exercise or he would have to see a psychologist. After much argument, a schedule was agreed upon, and his behaviour settled. A crisis had again been averted.

When I saw Philip in the clinic, he was in his mid-twenties and had just been appointed lecturer at a university. He was teaching accountancy. 'He has chosen well,' I thought, once I had learnt about his obsessionality.

His reason for the consultation: 'It is embarrassing to talk about it, but I have this strange idea in my head.' He hesitated.

'Yes, you can talk about it to me without any embarrassment,' I encouraged him.

'It is quite crazy ... sometimes I think I am going mad.'

'Yes.' I was being patient.

'I get this thought that the women I meet think I am staring at their chests ... I mean ... breasts. It is not really true ... er ... you see when you look at a woman, you look at the whole person, and that includes the breasts. It is not that I am staring at the breasts, but this thought comes into my head that this is what the woman is thinking. I then have to turn my eyes away. I can't even bear to look at her face.'

He said that he had always been somewhat shy and not very confident with girls. Girls, on the other hand, liked him. He was handsome, with a pleasant face and a nice smile. Above all, he had polite and endearing manners, which women found appealing. He went through his teenage years without dating, even though he was attracted to girls and was quite secure about his heterosexual orientation. In his university years, he made a few feeble attempts at going out with girls, but was uncomfortable and no lasting relationship ensued. His doctorate years were focused, with only hints of obsessionality – the occasional delayed assignment because of compulsive checking, some re-emergence of bedtime rituals when he was under stress – which did not interfere with his work. His colleagues did tell him to loosen up, but they liked his dependability – of course, his supervisor was delighted with his conscientiousness. Socialisation remained minimal and mainly with his extended family.

He was nearly 26 when he had his first meaningful relationship. Melanie was a gregarious and light-hearted person, full of humour and fun, complementing his seriousness and natural caution. He was attracted to her vivacity and the ease with which life's small decisions came to her.

'In her I could see the antithesis of myself. One could see that her shoulders were not drooped with the weight of the world ... She did not need to deliberate on which side of the bed she should get up from in the morning so as to allay the ghosts of the day.' He pondered on his obsessional nature – a kind of straitjacket for his personality. 'I sometimes wondered what she liked in me .... she was possibly seeking the opposite, just like myself. She was the best thing that happened to me. Mind you, she was not the most beautiful person you would come across, but that was not important.

'I remember the first time I had this strange thought. Melanie and I were at a party of a mutual friend – nothing special, just one of those Friday night affairs. I was introduced to this gorgeous girl – tall, attractive and flirtatious. What I most remember was the low cut of her blouse – her well-endowed breasts were almost bursting out. One couldn't help but stare at them – she seemed not to notice, as if she was used to men staring at her. I tried to strike up a conversation, but I was fumbling, and was relieved when she was distracted by someone else and moved on. A little later, Melanie came over.'

'"Who was that girl you were talking to?" she asked, almost jokingly.'

'"Oh! er ... Lisa ... she is a friend of the host."'

'"She's very pretty. I couldn't help noticing that you were staring at her breasts."'

'"I wasn't," I protested, rather weakly. "You see ... her cleavage ... never mind!" I was beginning to feel hot, and must have been red in the face.

'"It's all right," said Melanie. "You wouldn't be a man if you didn't. She's openly inviting it."'

'Melanie was obviously not feeling jealous, but I was decidedly uncomfortable. I know that my girlfriend is not – how should I put it … well endowed in the chest. I felt as if I had been rude, not to Lisa but to Melanie.'

'You mean small breasts,' I paraphrased.

'You see … I have difficulty even mentioning the word "breast". You may find that strange.'

'I am sorry for interrupting you.'

'Anyway … the thought did not leave me, although I argued with myself and tried to dismiss it. It kept nagging me that I had been so careless and had hurt Melanie's feelings.'

'So you thought you had hurt her feelings?'

'Maybe not. I do magnify such problems. She had reassured me.'

'Then …' I goaded him along.

'I carried on with my work. In the next few days, it was weighing less on me. I thought I had overcome it. Then suddenly …' He paused.

'Something must have brought the thought back.'

'It was this graduate student … again, rather busty, I must say. Decently dressed! She had come to me to discuss her assignment. Nothing inappropriate in that! This idea popped into my head that I was staring at her breasts. I tried to push it away, but the idea kept coming back. I was again red. I could not concentrate on what I was saying … just trying to keep my gaze away from her. I could not even look at her face … She must have thought I was a twit.'

This idea now became repetitive and spread. In the street

... at the train station ... in the lecture room – everywhere ... even during family gatherings. He had this troublesome idea in his head that he was staring at a woman's breast, and he would avert his eyes and not look at the woman. He would become nervous, and his concentration would falter. He tried his best to 'not think', but the harder he tried, the worse it would get. He was so troubled by the thought that he began to isolate himself, staying in his apartment and not venturing out except when he thought there would be few people about. The idea was no longer restricted to 'busty' women, but became associated with all women – even with his girlfriend.

'What really upset me was that it even happened with my grandmother. What would the old lady think of me if she knew what went on in my head? I was really ashamed of myself.'

Philip had clearly developed an obsession, and it was a symptom of obsessive compulsive disorder (OCD). I explained to him this idea had all the characteristics of an obsessional thought. This was not akin to saying that he was preoccupied with a thought. The thought had a 'subjective compulsiveness' about it – he could not help but think this thought even though he tried not to. It intruded into his consciousness, however unwanted or unacceptable it was. He tried to ignore or suppress it but without success. It was his own thought – a product of his own mind – but a part of the mind over which he could not exercise control. It was an alien thought – one that was his own but that he did not wish to have. It was senseless – it had no implication that he was rude or lecherous – and he recognised its senselessness.

I tried to reassure him. I could unequivocally allay his fear that he was not going mad or psychotic. 'The main distinction between your mind and someone who is psychotic is that you know what you are thinking is wrong or unwanted, but you cannot help it. The psychotic mind is not aware of its deviance. The technical term for that is insight – madness equates with lack of insight. Your problem is quite the reverse – it is the presence, indeed overdevelopment, of insight that torments you. You are troubled by an excess of sanity, in some ways. There is no chance that you will begin to stare at women's breasts or reach out to grab them.'

'But why breasts? Why did it have to be breasts? My trouble is that more than half the world's population has breasts – I have no escape.'

I had no simple answer to this question. Breasts on a female form are very important organs indeed. While men have breasts that are structurally identical to those of women, breasts are generally identified with women and are important symbols of sexuality and fertility. Philip was not troubled by men's breasts – I reminded him that even men had breasts, but they remained rudimentary. The development of breasts in girls is emblematic of pubescence and sexual maturity, and the sight of breasts is sexually arousing for men. The nipples are sexually sensitive for women, thereby increasing their sexual significance. Philip informed me that pre-pubescent girls did not produce the same reaction, although his eyes were now more keenly aware of the rudiments of breast development on young girls' chests.

Philip's question had a self-reference, but there was a broader question: why had the human female developed permanently enlarged breasts? It is a question that has puzzled evolutionary theorists since our primate cousins, such as the chimpanzee and gorilla, do not have this characteristic. You are typically not able to distinguish a female ape or monkey from a male by the size of the breast. While the female ape's breast does engorge during pregnancy and lactation, it recedes to a flat appearance once the lactation is over. Most anthropologists believe that human female breasts are sexual signals, much like the plumage of the peacock.

Desmond Morris, author of the popular book *The Naked Ape*,[2] argued that human females developed enlarged breasts because of their bipedalism. One defining feature of humans is that they walk upright on two feet. With the attainment of this characteristic, sexual encounters between humans became face-to-face. In our primate cousins, the presentation of the female buttocks is an erotic display to the male to provoke sexual interest. In a frontal encounter, this was not an effective strategy, and nature favoured the development of a persistently enlarged female breast, in what is referred to as 'self-mimicry'. Other writers have referred to the breasts as the equivalents of female genitalia.[3]

Do large breasts really offer a sexual advantage to women, thereby explaining their selective selection in evolution? There are a few problems with this theory. Charles Darwin believed that it was in the interest of survival of a species for all women to mate and bear children. For this reason, in the animal kingdom, males are the ones to develop elaborate sexual displays rather than females − contrast the magnificence of the peacock with the peahen, or the lion with the lioness. What was different about humans that the female sexual characteristics were so prominent? An attempt at answering this has come from socio-biology, according to which traits survive and prosper in species because they offer a sexual advantage. It is accepted by this theory that males have a survival advantage in terms of passing on their genes by having multiple partners, whereas females, because of their great investment in pregnancy and lactation, increase their reproductive advantage by being relatively chaste and enticing a man to support them over the longer term. This, according to sociobiology, is the 'domestic-bliss strategy' of the female hominid, and big breasts are a tool in this strategy. Breasts are seen as signals that alert the male to the female most likely to successfully raise his progeny. Breasts are primarily made up of fat cells, and females better able to build up and maintain fat have greater reserve for pregnancy and lactation, thereby increasing their reproductive attractiveness.

There are a number of assumptions in the sociobiological explanation that might not be true. There is no evidence that busty women are more likely to gain and keep a mate than their flatter-chested sisters. Nor is there evidence that breast size relates to reproductive potential. Many other hypotheses in relation to the selection of sexual traits lack scientific evidence. The assumption of female dependency for survival on male partners has been questioned by some anthropologists.[4]

I tried to explain to Philip that we essentially do not know why larger breasts were attractive to men, but there was little doubt that at least in most Western societies, this was indeed the case. Perhaps it was simply that during the hunter-gatherer period of human existence, good nutritional reserve conferred greater survival potential and therefore reproductive advan-tage, and large breasts were emblematic of that. Whatever their origin – and Philip was not interested in the evolution of these protuberances – there was agreement that in modern society, breasts were sexual organs.

The cultural attitude to breasts reveals considerable ambivalence, and this may be at the root of Philip's problems. Many prehistoric cultures had an open attitude to exposure of breasts by women. This had continued to modern times in certain societies. Philip was familiar with the indigenous Australians – the Aborigines – in whom the exposure of the female breast did not have the same taboo as among white Australians. Yet Europeans were more relaxed about it than Islamic societies. Breasts as sexual objects had been exploited by artists through the centuries. The portraits of Venus were fine examples of this. The prohibition against breast exposure was relaxed to varying degrees in certain settings. Philip avoided going to the beach altogether. Not only did the bikini accentuate the breasts but also his favourite Bondi Beach not uncommonly had bare-breasted women soaking up the sun for a quick tan.

'Perhaps staring would be acceptable there, but I would still be tormented,' he explained his position.

'These women exposing their breasts are trying to assert their equality with men – a kind of feminism with a sun-drenched appeal,' I suggested. 'They are suggesting that their breasts are not sexual organs … but I think it is a weak attempt as it is restricted to the beach, and most would baulk at doing the same in a restaurant or on the street.'

Philip was assured that he was not 'crazy', but could this be a sexual deviation? 'Am I some sort of pervert to think these thoughts?' was a question I suspected he wanted to put to me. I pre-empted it.

'The obsession does not imply that you have developed a sexual deviation either,' I told him. 'There is such a thing as a breast fetish, but it is quite the opposite of what you suffer. These men – they are always men – prefer large breasts as objects of desire, sometimes exclusively so. There can be variations on the theme – there may be a preference for puffy areolae, or long or thick nipples, and even lactating or bouncy breasts. The preference for large breasts is more a cultural trait rather than a fetish, but it is sad to see young girls wishing to enhance their breasts artificially to make themselves more attractive to men. There is a whole industry out there based on this notion of the attractiveness of big breasts. The Pamela Andersons of the world recognise this, and use it or allow themselves to be used to obtain material gain. The bottom line is that a fetishist derives pleasure from such an encounter. For you, the very thought of looking at a breast is a torment. You have a classic case of OCD.'

Philip saw me on a few occasions. He sincerely wanted treatment for his obsession. Equally important to him was to understand why he had developed this particular symptom. He believed that unless he understood it, he would not be able to conquer it. Being internet savvy and having access to a university library, he had a vast amount of information available to him. He was struggling to put it together. When I broached the idea of treatment with a drug, he was quite dismissive. 'It would be like putting a patch on a big hole,' he argued. 'Not only would it be ugly, but also sooner or later the hole would become bigger than the patch could cover.'

'You have had some obsessionality from an early age,' I tried to explain. I had been able to interview his mother to put together the case for this. There had been times in his life when the scale had almost tipped in favour of obsessive compulsive symptoms. His night-time rituals of folding his clothes were early markers of compulsive behaviour. His checking behaviour, and his preoccupation with exercise, also suggested the same tendency.

'We do distinguish between obsessions and compulsions. Your repetitive and unwelcome idea is an obsession. In other cases, one can have repetitive images or impulses. Compulsions on the other hand involve actions – actions that you do not want but cannot resist. Checking your arithmetic assignment twice was acceptable, but if you were driven to check it seven times, that is a compulsion.'

'There were times when I did check my assignment three times even when I knew there were no errors. Was that a compulsion?'

'It is hard to know where to draw the line. One characteristic I use is that of senselessness. When an objective outsider begins to see that the repetition is senseless, it is a problem. Another indicator is when the repetition in fact prevents you from actually being able to complete the task. Sometimes, the task is repeated a certain number of times – often a magical number such as seven is picked – with the belief that if the number of repetitions do not meet this criterion, something devastating would happen.'

'It never happened to me quite in this manner. I did think that if my assignment was not free of errors, I would fail – that is possibly not the devastation you mean.'

'Often it is the death of a family member – something unrelated, suggesting a magical occurrence. There is often this magical quality about compulsions, which shows how primitive the mind can be in such cases.'

'But the problem I now have is what you called an obsession.' Philip brought the discussion back to himself. 'It is an idea, not an action. I must say, I do turn my eyes away from the bosom – that could be a compulsion.'

'I would not regard that as a compulsion,' I replied. 'It does not have the repetitive quality about it. In any case, there is no need to be too particular about this distinction. Most investigators believe that all compulsions occur in response to obsessions, although this can be disputed. Certainly, you need a thought before an action, although that thought could be an impulse. The diagnosis is the same – obsessive-compulsive disorder (OCD) – whether you have an obsession or a compulsion or both. Most people would have both at some stage of their illness, although one or the other may predominate.'

'About my obsession ... why now? Why this peculiar obsession?'

Reasons certain mental phenomena happen are buried within the layers of the mind. A scientist could not but argue that there must be a reason, or a set of reasons, in response to Philip's questions. This was one of Sigmund Freud's major contributions to psychology: he forcefully argued that mental symptoms do not arise from a void, but are consequences of the turmoil deep in the mind – in the unconscious. Freud was a master at uncovering those causes, but the revelation could take months or years and there was no formal proof that the supposed revelation was indeed the truth! No doubt I was not going to supply Philip with a quick answer to such a difficult question.

I did have some hypotheses regarding the origin of Philip's obsessions. It started with a certain characteristic of his brain function, something attributable to his genes. It is well recognised that OCD can run in families, and identical (monozygotic) twins are more likely to have a concordance of the disorder, i.e. it is more likely that both twins either do or do not have the disorder compared with non-identical (dizygotic) twins. No single gene has been identified for the disorder – and not for lack of searching by various groups around the world! It seems that OCD is not likely to be related to abnormality of a single gene. This is not surprising, considering that obsessionality as a personality feature *per se* is such a common manifestation in society, and OCD is said to affect 2–3 per cent of the population, at least in its milder form. Such common traits have multiple genetic determinants. It is more likely that OCD is related to the coming together of a number of genes, each with a small effect, much like the hand of an unlucky player in a card game. Of course, the fact that your parents carry those particular genes increases your chances of getting them, explaining the family history of OCD. Interestingly, this family history may include other disorders such as Tourette's syndrome, anorexia nervosa or even disorders like abnormal hair pulling (trichotillomania). Since recent advances have given us the ability to examine the entire genome for aberrations, it might not be long until we discover a string of genes that predispose an individual to OCD.

'Predispose is the operative word,' I explained to Philip. 'Having a particular set of genes would still not mean that you have OCD. These genes would cause a certain kind of brain to develop, which then interacts with special features in your environment to produce the disorder.'

'What is that kind of brain, and can you tell if I have such a brain?' This was a perfectly valid question, I thought. I could send Philip for an MRI scan,[5] but I was unlikely to see any abnormality on such a scan. The MRI is excellent for studying the structure of the brain, which is normal in patients with OCD. Their brains do not look different from those of healthy individuals. The older neurological literature refers to the development of obsessive compulsive symptoms in patients who suffered from encephalitis lethargica. On post-mortem examination, these patients had lesions in the basal ganglia: the caudate, putamen and globus pallidus, clumps of brain cells that sit just in the middle of the brain and act as relay stations for the processing of information relating to movement, thought and emotion. Obsessive compulsive symptoms are also associated with Tourette's syndrome, Sydenham's chorea, carbon monoxide poisoning, and other disorders in which basal ganglia are known to be involved.

A somewhat more useful scan might be a PET scan,[6] which examines the metabolic rate in different brain regions. Abnormalities in metabolic rates have been described in OCD patients, in particular increased activity in the orbitofrontal cortex – the part of the frontal lobes that sits above the eye sockets – as well as the caudate nucleus.

The orbitofrontal cortex appears to be a critical area in OCD. It is the region of the brain that integrates emotional information and relates it to positive or negative reward. It therefore biases the choice for or against a particular emotional stimulus. This would help facilitate decisions when faced with complex or plentiful options by providing information that favours appropriate choices. Those choices that are rewarding would be enhanced, and the ones associated with punishment or negative consequences would be inhibited. In this context, it is interesting to entertain the possibility that 'gut feeling' relates to orbitofrontal cortical activity. When a formerly rewarding option that is no longer rewarding is later presented, this brain region is likely to be involved in suppressing its selection. In this manner, the orbitofrontal cortex maintains a representation of reward history of the individual and modifies former reward representations that may have currently become disadvantageous. The actual decision-making – to accept or reject a particular choice – is not made by the orbitofrontal but by the dorsolateral prefrontal cortex (DLPFC), the part of the frontal lobe that lies on the side of the brain. In very simple, well-structured decisions, the DLPFC would require little influence from the orbitofrontal cortex as such decisions would probably not involve much emotional processing. Conversely, decisions that rely predominantly upon prior reward history – whether such decisions led to a positive or negative consequence in the past – probably engage the orbitofrontal cortex quite actively, with little DLPFC involvement. This is supported, in part, by the fact that damage to the orbitofrontal cortex has been classically associated with abnormal decision-making in daily life even though the individual retains the ability to make the correct choices. Such individuals become impulsive and make bad choices, based on immediate gratification. They may lose the inhibitions normally expected during social intercourse.

Philip's situation was quite the opposite of that seen in the sociopathic behaviour of a person with orbitofrontal lesions – the likes of Stephen we met in chapter 6. One could speculate that Philip's orbitofrontal cortex was probably overactive. This has indeed been observed in the PET scans of OCD patients, especially in the outer part of the orbitofrontal cortex which is more sensitive to the negative consequences of actions. This overactivity may imbue an otherwise neutral idea or action with such negative emotional energy that it continues to repetitively trouble the mind, not permitting the other frontal brain regions to close the action by a decision. This was one possible scenario for the brain basis for Philip's obsession: an innocuous viewing of the breasts of an attractive woman, which for the average individual would be a passing gaze, had aroused such deep negative emotion that it had become impossible to obliterate.

'Let me put this to you. You say that you are careful and check your work a few times. Now suppose the assignment you are about to submit is really important – say, your job depends on it. You are likely to check this even more, and perhaps go over it in your mind right through the night and be unable to sleep. You will not be able to calmly put it aside and not worry about it.'

'I agree with you. Its importance – or the possibility of an adverse outcome – will make the situation worse.'

'Now suppose your very life, or the life of a loved one, depended upon the accuracy of information in the assignment.'

'That would send me round the bend! I can see what you are driving at – the greater the charge of emotional energy, the stronger the need to repeat – at least for me that is true.'

'The OCD brain unfortunately attaches the same emotional

energy to an idea or an image that for most purposes is rather banal or inconsequential. In your case, looking at the breasts signals to your brain that some devastation will occur, and your rational mind is unable to overcome this powerful signal. The energy has been attached to what should otherwise be a relatively neutral idea, possibly because your orbitofrontal cortex is overactive.'

Philip would have liked some proof that the orbitofrontal cortex was indeed overactive. The problem was that interpreting an individual PET scan is fraught with difficulties, as the values are relative rather than absolute. PET scanning is expensive, as each scan costs more than $2000. I would have performed the scan if some invasive treatment such as surgery was being planned. I remembered a previous patient of mine who, after having failed many years of medical treatment, was treated with surgical lesions in the white matter adjacent to the orbitofrontal cortex. She did remarkably well, considering the debilitating OCD she had suffered for many years, and her PET scans showed improvement following the surgery.[7] Philip did not go for a PET after assessing the costs and any potential benefit.

'If there is a genetic basis, how do you relate that to the PET scan abnormality?' asked Philip.

'You indeed have a scientific mind — many investigators would like to ask this question, but unfortunately the data are not yet available to answer it. Genes are of course important in brain development. The human genome has about 30 000 genes — perhaps less. What is significant is that about half these genes are involved in some way with the nervous system. There are two unknowns: we do not yet have precise knowledge of the genes involved in various aspects of brain development, although this knowledge is fast accumulating, and we do not know which genes are important for OCD.'

'So I have a brain, which, by virtue of the genes inherited, makes me a sitting duck.'

'Vulnerable yes, but a sitting duck maybe not! Genes may be the script or the alphabet, but the development of the brain is a dynamic process reflecting the interaction of these genes with the environment.'

'That environment was provided by my parents, just like my genes. It seems fair to blame them for my condition.'

'That would be an error, in my opinion.' I tried to defend the hapless parents. 'It is true that your genes come from your parents, but they never intended to pass on the wrong set of genes. Some of this is a shuffle by nature, like a deck of cards – there is no one to blame for a weak hand. Your parents do create the environment you grow up in, but the environment is also influenced by the child. There is an old saying that the children bring up their parents. The environment your brother grew up in was not the same as your own, since he influenced his environment just as you did yours.'

'It was only in jest – I do not blame my parents. They come as a package, you see – you can't just pick out the good bits.' Philip was philosophical about it.

'Coming back to the symptom – why this obsession? Was that not your question? I am afraid we are coming into specu- lative territory. More accurately, I have to borrow from psycho- dynamic theorists – psychoanalysts, as you might call them. Some of these theories originated from Pierre Janet,[8] a French psychologist who in fact pre-dated Freud by a few years. Some even regard him as the father of psychoanalysis. The basis of the obsession is a conflict. In your case, the overt conflict is your attractiveness towards this busty woman and your need to remain loyal to your girlfriend, whom you care for. This conflict leads to psychological tension,[9] which is relieved by a process Janet calls displacement. You are reinvesting the mental energy into the idea of staring at the breasts, something less troublesome than being disloyal to your girlfriend and from which you can avert your eyes.'

'That's a neat explanation. It makes sense to me in some ways, although the thought of disloyalty never crossed my mind.'

'That is the premise of psychodynamics – such conflicts are played out below the surface, in the subterranean space of the unconscious. Psychoanalysis brings it to conscious awareness so that the conflict can be worked through.'

'Now that you have provided the explanation – if it is true, will my obsession gradually wane and disappear? Since I am now aware of its devious message, does my mind still need it?'

'I'm afraid, just "telling" you may not be enough. A psychoanalyst attempts to make you "discover" it through a process of analysis. You now have intellectual insight into the problem, yet what you really need, according to this theory, is emotional insight. That can be a long and arduous process. If you achieve it, your problem will lose its power over you, but there is no guarantee.'

'I am not an impatient person, but I need relief faster than that. Is there something else I can do?'

I agreed that Philip was not impatient. His personality showed the signs of compulsiveness – he was controlled, reserved, punctual, fastidious, reliable and boring. This is how he had always been – his character was hard-wired in his brain. Freud would certainly call him an anal-retentive character,[10] although I find it difficult to relate personalities to erotic body parts, and therefore did not raise this with him.

'My recommendation is to combine drug treatment with behaviour therapy,' I said. 'I think that drugs will offer you relief in the short term, but for the effects to last, behaviour therapy may offer an advantage.'

I was aware of Philip's resistance to drug treatment. Why intelligent people often find it difficult to reconcile drug treatment with a mental problem is difficult for me to understand. Richard (in chapter 7) had the same resistance to this idea. I have spent much of my professional life explaining to patients the molecular workings of the brain.

One of the first modern advances in neuroscience was the discovery of neural transmission: that nerve cells talk to each other with the help of molecules called neurotransmitters. These discoveries have been the basis for many Nobel prizes, and are established dogma. We also know that a single neuron is in itself quite dumb. No thought or emotion ever originated from a single neuron. It is only when a group of neurons connect with each other as a functional unit that any semblance of mental activity originates. It is not hard to understand why drugs that alter the level of these traversing chemicals will affect mental processes. Perhaps it is the fear that the drug may be too blunt an instrument to achieve fine tuning of the brain. Arguably, any defect in transmission, if it is the basis for obsessions, must be fairly restricted in the brain, whereas any drug will not discriminate between normal and abnormal neuronal circuits. This may or may not be true. There is considerable plasticity in the brain, such that it is able to partially repair itself, given the right encouragement. Could it be that the drugs are that sort of encouragement, and actions on some chemical receptors are one means of providing it? I did not have a clear explanation for the 'real' mechanism by which drugs acted, and had to leave many blanks unfilled. I could allay the fears that these drugs were addictive, however, at least by the classic measures of habituation (an urge to take the drug for its positive effect), tolerance (a need for increasing doses to produce the same effect) and withdrawal (the development of withdrawal symptoms upon ceasing its use – the body complaining about missing its effects).

Philip knew a great deal about serotonin. It has come to be popularly regarded as the mood molecule, but this was not how it was discovered. Scientists in the Cleveland Clinic first discovered this substance in the serum in 1948,[11] and showed that it caused the contraction of smooth muscle organs – hence the name sero-tonin (i.e. a substance in the serum that increases muscle tone). Italian scientists, around the same time, isolated the substance from the gut. The purified substance was called 5-hydroxytryptamine (5HT) and it is the same as serotonin. It was later shown to be present in the brain, and its structure resembled that of LSD, the psychedelic drug abused at parties. The cells that contain serotonin in the brain are present in the brain stem but send their projections to much of the brain, thereby playing a regulatory role in many functions. Serotonin has been shown to have a role in the regulation of anger, aggression, body temperature, mood, sleep, vomiting, sexuality and appetite. There is a general notion that in such disorders as depression and OCD, there is a deficiency of serotonin, and increasing its level at the site of the receptors would have a therapeutic effect. When one examines the variety of receptors that serotonin acts on, this appears to be too simple an approach to a complex system. There are at least eight subtypes of serotonin receptors in the brain with different functions. All drugs shown to be helpful for OCD do, however, have the property of increasing the levels of serotonin at the receptor site. How this translates into anti-obsessional properties is unknown, but one can speculate that this modulates the activity of certain brain circuits.

Serotonin is present in certain fruits and vegetables, but the body's serotonin is largely manufactured from tryptophan, an amino acid found in many proteins. Ingested serotonin cannot cross the blood–brain barrier to enter the brain, but tryptophan can, from which serotonin can be manufactured in the brain. Tryptophan has consequently been used to help with sleep.

Was Philip's brain deficient in serotonin? There was no way of knowing for sure. Theoretically, one could use the PET scan to measure aspects of serotonin transmission in the brain. One could use a radiotracer to measure the level of a certain type of serotonin receptors. Another radiotracer can show the level of activity of the serotonin transporter, the molecule responsible for taking up the serotonin released in the synapse back into the neuron. The difficulty in the clinical setting is that these measurements are still not applicable to individual cases and, even when applied to groups, only build an incomplete picture of the real state of serotonin function, which itself is dynamic and adaptable.

'Unfortunately, the technology we have, while very

advanced, is still unable to give us a snapshot of the serotonin in your brain. We have to go with a presumption,' I tried to explain to him.

'But what if my serotonin levels are normal? Is that possible?'

'I have no way of knowing that. It is entirely possible – we know that serotonin transmission may be abnormal even when the levels are normal. This has to relate to receptors, uptake and other things. Don't forget, abnormality in serotonin may not be the only explanation for OCD – most likely, it isn't.'

'What would happen if my serotonin levels are normal but I take a drug to increase them further? Could that not be counter-productive?'

I had no informed answer to this question. All patients treated with drugs to alter serotonin in the brain suffer side effects, presumably related to altered levels in the brain as well as the body, especially the gut. Only some show an improvement in their disorder. It is impossible to pick with any certainty the ones who will.

'If you do not try the drug, we will never know' was my considered response.

Philip agreed to take a drug – 'Only as a trial,' as he put it – with the agreement that he could discontinue it if he wished. When I explained to him the large number of drugs that we could choose from, but that I did not know which one was best for him, he was not impressed. He had picked another hole in the knowledge base. All the drugs shared one property – that of blocking the serotonin transporter to varying degrees – but differed subtly in their other properties. Moreover, each individual body handles these drugs differently in terms of absorption, metabolism, excretion etc. For the individual, it was a hit-and-miss strategy. Philip was started on sertraline, a drug belonging to the group of serotonin-specific reuptake inhibitors (SSRIs), with the dose gradually increased over a few weeks. He did this while he awaited a consultation with a behaviour therapist.

It was three months since the initiation of the drug. Philip had not yet started the behavioural treatment, and was feeling unsure about it. His obsession had not been cured, but the intensity of the emotion associated with the thought was definitely reduced. When the thought of staring at someone's breasts entered his mind, he could reason with himself and dismiss the thought for the moment. He had therefore become less avoidant of contacts with women and no longer isolated himself. He could face a woman and talk to her in a social interaction. He was more relaxed in the company of his girlfriend. His experience with the drug had not been too negative. He had experienced some nausea initially, but this settled in a couple of weeks. He noted some tiredness and 'laziness', but was willing to pay this price for the benefit that had ensued. I persuaded him to follow through with the behaviour therapy to produce a lasting change. It was satisfying to know that, once Philip started seeing a clinical psychologist for this behaviour therapy, there would be at least one other person subjected to the same difficult questions on how the brain worked.

Philip maintained his medication for two years, while also continuing the behaviour therapy. His obsession was now a memory of the past – he felt that he had mastered it. He slowly lowered the dose of the medication, then stopped it completely. There was no recurrence. He had learnt the techniques to challenge any aberrant thoughts in his head. He ended his last consultation with me with a thoughtful admission: 'I realise that this could happen again, but I am now equipped to curb the turbulence of any molecules of serotonin. I also accept that the medication blunted serotonin's charge for this to happen.'

9

Lord Nelson's ghost

The Most Noble Lord Horatio Nelson, Viscount and Baron Nelson, of the Nile and of Burnham Thorpe in the County of Norfolk, Knight of the Most Honourable Order of the Bath, Vice Admiral of the White Squadron of the Fleet, Commander in Chief of his Majesty's Ships and Vessels in the Mediterranean, Duke of Bronte in Sicily, Knight Grand Cross of the Sicilian Order of St Ferdinand and of Merit, Member of the Ottoman Order of the Crescent, Knight Grand Commander of the Order of St Joachim.

The Naval Chronicle, p. 223[1]

The journey through Julian's problems proved to be tortuous. He was sent to me for the treatment of depression following a car accident that resulted in severe damage to his left arm. 'It was a mangled wreck,' he informed me. The surgeon had no choice but to amputate the arm just above the elbow. 'My girlfriend wept when she saw me. I wept with her, something I had not done since the accident … I am a tough sort of fellow, or so I always thought. This thing throws you off, doc. You don't expect it to happen to you … Maybe it's about being young. You think these things happen only to other unfortunate people.'

Julian was a thoughtful man of 23 who had recently completed his university studies and had entered junior management in a private company. He was charming and sensitive, a New Age man brimming with promise. His mother, who had emigrated to Australia from England, had struggled to single-handedly give him the best opportunities in life. She had prepared him for adversity, he said, and the plenty he had experienced in his early employment had seemed to him as a gift not to be taken for granted. She had also taught him to be tolerant, not a little by her own example. The devastating loss of the arm had not initially been the apocalypse that his friends had feared. But things had begun to change. It was now two months since the accident, and the hue of his world was a distinct grey. He had not slept for days, and his clothes hung loosely over his slight frame, suggesting a loss of weight. He had not gone back to work since the accident. I assumed a severely damaged sense of self, a trauma to which there could be no other response but a withdrawal within. I thought I understood his depression. I sympathised with his loss.

His response took me by surprise. He admitted to the depression, the 'greying of his soul' as he put it, but it was not a response to the loss he had suffered. 'I have come to terms with that, incredible as it may seem. I have begun to see myself as a one-handed person, and a complete one at that. I had a dream last night in which I had one arm. It didn't faze me. Dr Sachdev, it's not the loss of the arm, but the pain. This pain is incredible, and I am fed up with all the drugs that the Pain Clinic has given me.'

I had been informed about the pain by the physician who had been treating Julian. The physician told me that pain in the stump was not uncommon after an amputation, and the various drugs they had tried one by one to alleviate the pain had been unhelpful. In general, the result had been a thumbs-down from Julian. 'It would have been OK if they had been able to put me to sleep around the clock. But the drugs could not manage that.' The drugs numbed him more than they numbed the pain. The physician had gone on to inject anaesthetic drugs into the stump, with partial but temporary relief. He had gone back to the surgeon seeking a cure for the pain, and the surgeon had suggested that perhaps surgery to further shorten the limb might help. He argued that the pain was caused by inflamed or overactive nerves at the site of the stump – these nerves formed little growths or neuromas in some cases. Shortening the stump would remove these neuromas and give a clean ending to these nerves. Julian was not convinced by the argument that the shortening would somehow help, and the surgeon had been noncommittal about the chances of improvement.

I explained to Julian that he had been sent to see me to explore possible psychological causes of the pain. It was not hard to understand why this might be the case. Pain was, after all, a mental phenomenon and can be modified by psychological factors. We talked of psychic pain in a metaphorical sense, and that such pain can be felt as pain in the body as well. Hypnotism has been used both to alleviate pain and to produce it. Pain can also be a symptom of depression. Was Julian's pain the manifestation of his depression? I set about exploring this possibility. It was not an attempt to explain the pain in its entirety but to attribute to the mental state an amplifying role. It was then that Julian revealed the true nature of his problem. The pain was not in the stump of his amputated limb.

'Now, how can I explain this to you, Dr Sachdev, without sounding crazy? Ever since the amputation, I have felt as if I have not really lost my arm. It is still there, hanging by my side, stiff and unbending. When I look at it, I only see this prosthesis in its place, but when I close my eyes, my left hand and arm are back, just as they were before their removal. And it hurts!'

Julian expected me to be taken by surprise, even fall off my chair! He was astonished by my equanimity. His admission, in fact, produced no surprise at all. What he was describing was the experience of a phantom limb – not uncommon at all. The majority of individuals who lose a limb experience this feeling of the continuing presence of the limb. In most cases, this feeling gradually fades away over the following days and weeks. In as many as 30 per cent of cases, it persists for a long time, possibly years and decades. No one was therefore likely to consider him crazy. I gave him the example of Lord Nelson, the revered British admiral who led the British navy in the Napoleonic wars and was credited with the decisive defeat of Napoleon in the Battle of the Nile and the Battle of Trafalgar. In 1797 he led an expedition to conquer Santa Cruz de Tenerife, a Spanish city in the Canary Islands. Not only was the mission unsuccessful but also he was shot in the arm with a musket ball and fractured his humerus bone in many places. He had to undergo an amputation of his right arm; he later referred to the stump as 'my fin'. He experienced the sensation of phantom limb and even had severe pain in his limb. He was so taken by this ghostly sensation that he considered it proof that there must be a soul that survived after the body was annihilated,[2] just as the ghost of the limb had survived its removal.

'Well, that's a relief. It seems I am in good company. All this while, I have not told anyone about it, not even my mother. It has been my secret, but a difficult one to keep. I am not one to believe in ghosts, but the ghost of my lost hand is always with me. And it is a painful ghost. The Lord Nelson story is a wonderful one. The Battle of Trafalgar is my favourite battle in history. By the way, October 21 is next week, and when I was in England, they used to call it Trafalgar Day.'

'What a coincidence! Your phantom limb may well be Lord Nelson's ghost!'

Julian had not told the physician about his experience of the phantom limb, little realising that this would not have surprised him in the least. Phantoms have been described in the medical literature since the time of S. Weir Mitchell's[3] descriptions in the late nineteenth century and are accepted by physicians as common and perfectly sane outcomes of amputation. The explanations of phantom limbs have varied, depending upon the background and biases of the proponents of the theories. As a phenomenon, it is generally regarded as an illusion, a mistaken perception, and the individual experiencing it recognises it to be just that. The individual is not deluded or crazy, which would be the case if he actually believed that the limb was present. Illusions, like mistaking a rope in the dark for a snake, are often brought about by an ambiguity of stimuli. In the case of phantom limbs, the commonly held theory is that the nerves fibres cut during the amputation of the limb continue to provide sensory input to the brain, providing that ambiguity of stimuli usually required for an illusion. Unlike the snake illusion, however, the phantom experience persists despite clear knowledge of its illusory nature. Visual feedback, while clearly informing the brain that the limb is absent, does not correct the illusion. Sensory input from the nerve endings also does not seem to be necessary for the phantom to persist. If the stump is injected with a local anaesthetic, or the sensory nerves in the stump are cut, the feeling persists. Even blocking the sensory input at the level of the spinal cord is not a 'cure' of the phantom limb.

Not surprisingly, this experience provides a fertile basis for psychoanalytical speculation. Classic Freudian thought views this as a non-acceptance of loss, a form of denial that operates at the unconscious level. A man recovering from a life-threatening heart attack starts exercising to prepare himself for the city-to-surf race he had long been planning to run, even though the cardiologist warns him of the danger. That is the classical example of denial in psychodynamic terms. A widow mourns the loss of her husband by keeping his study untouched, even putting a fresh glass of fruit juice on his desk every morning. She feels a strong sense of his presence in the house, and is unable to discard any of his clothes, while acknowledging that he is dead. Could the phantom limb be a similar kind of denial of a tragic loss? Amputees not uncommonly report dreams in which they see an intact body – could this simply be an 'awake' dream? Many individuals with a phantom limb report that the limb becomes smaller with time as it telescopes into the stump. Could this be a Freudian compromise between the id and the ego: a psychological adjustment to the loss and its denial?[4] On the surface, this seems perfectly plausible, the mind tricking itself to preserve a sense of wholeness and continuity. The trouble is that this explanation is not supported by any evidence. Julian was not your prototypical 'denying' sort of individual. His history was one of brutal acceptance of reality,

which included the fact of his lost limb. He was not project-
ing an image of wholeness to the world. On the contrary, he
had hidden this illusion from everyone – even his mother –
and had projected himself as a one-handed individual keen to
carry on with life. To what purpose the denial, if denial it was?
And denial to whom? He was not denying it to the world, nor
was he denying it to himself. You will agree that there is some
strangeness in this explanation.

More contemporary views of the phantom limb have
been provided by Dr Ronald Melzack[5] of McGill University
in Montreal and Dr V. S. Ramachandran[6] of the University of
California at San Diego. I tried to explain these to Julian.

Dr Melzack was struck by the 'quality of reality' of the
phantom limb experience. He argued that this must be due to
the same brain processes that operate when the body is intact.
We experience our body as a unity, which is not dependent
upon the sensory input, although such input may influence our
experience of the body. He therefore argued that the explanation of the phantom experience must be sought in the brain.
He proposed a network of neurons in the brain, which is widespread and forms what he called a 'neuro-matrix'. This receives
inputs from the various body parts and forms a characteristic
pattern of activity that he called the 'neurosignature', which
underlies how we perceive our bodies. Interruption of input
from one body part, such as an amputated arm, is not sufficient
to alter the neurosignature – the feeling of the presence of the
limb therefore persists. Hence the phantom!

This made sense to Julian. The limb did seem real to him,
although when he looked at the stump, he could hardly believe
what he saw. He tried on an artificial limb a few times, and

the ghost – er, the phantom – enveloped it, 'as if to make it its own'.

Julian found it strange that sensory input did not seem really necessary for us to experience our limbs. This is an intriguing scientific question as well. The questions Dr Ramachandran rightly poses are: how does the brain generate an image of the body, and why does this image persist in the form of a phantom even when a limb has been removed? The image we have of our bodies is usually a stable percept that the brain generates by integrating information from a variety of inputs. We can refer to this stable percept as our 'body image'. The different sources may sometimes provide discrepant information. However, the brain must quickly reconcile this in order to support a stable schema that can guide behaviour. There is no room for a vacillating, now-this-now-that, image, even if this requires a piece of information that does not fit. Dr Ramachandran and his colleague William Hirstein[7] put it as follows: 'In doing this, the organism is making a bet, that if multiple sources of information concur in their verdict, then a single piece of discrepant information can safely be regarded as noise, or as a temporary malfunction of the sensory system which can be ignored.'

In the case of Julian's phantom limb, the discrepant input was coming from his eyes. There were many other sources of information that supported the presence of a limb.[8] We arguably start with a genetically determined image of the body, which is present from childhood. Then, of course, one has had this limb for a long time and remembers it well. There are these 'somatic memories' of a limb, which will not go away just because the limb is not present any more. There may be a contribution by the sensations from the stump with nerve endings that often form little balls of fibres or neuromas. These sources of information work towards creating the percept of the hand even after an amputation has occurred. The visual input now says that the hand is no longer there. Normal sensations from the skin and joints of the hand are also not present. The more recent memory of the severance of the hand is telling the brain that the limb is no longer present. However, in many cases, the brain ignores these discrepant inputs as noise that must be suppressed so that its originally stable 'body image' is not disturbed.

'It seems to me that my brain is a stubborn creature,' remarked Julian.

I had to agree with Julian that consistency was important for brain function. The brain has evolved to provide us with a consistent view of the world and of ourselves within it. It has evolved thinking that an individual has two hands, and this is implicit in the way the two cerebral hemispheres keep tabs on each other. As Robert exemplified so well in chapter 2, the brain comprises two halves – the right and left hemisphere – that are interconnected through a large bundle of fibres called the corpus collosum and smaller bundles called the commissures. For motor and sensory functions, each half is essentially connected to the other half of the body, so that the left hemisphere talks to the right hand and receives messages from it and vice versa. However, when sensations pour in from the right hand, some of them are sent to the right hemisphere as well, to regions that are a mirror image of the left hemisphere. It is the same with motor commands. The cortex in the right hemisphere becomes active when a command needs to be sent to the left hand, but minor activity is also detected on the other side. This may help maintain the illusion of two hands even when one is absent.

The brain's stubbornness has its limits. The brain is also quite plastic, as we now recognise. In fact, at the physiological level, the brain is making compensations and adapting rapidly. Dr Ramachandran suggested a few mechanisms. We know that there is a representation of the body in the brain, such that body regions like the thumb, arms, face, lips etc. send sensations to particular regions of the cortex. This is referred to as a 'somatotopic representation',[9] and enables us to localise sensations to any particular spot on the body. This schema has been well mapped out from the days of Wilder Penfield, the brilliant Canadian neurosurgeon. There exists a narrow strip of cortex in the brain that extends from the top and goes down on both sides, which is called the sensory cortex. Penfield showed that stimulation of this part of the brain produced sensations in different body regions with a distinct topography such that the body could be mapped on to the cortex in the form of a 'sensory homunculus'. The shape of the homunculus shows that it is a deformed creature with a rather large face, with prominent lips and big hands, suggesting that the brain devotes relatively large portions of the cortex to sensations from these regions. No wonder the lips and the finger tips are acutely sensitive to touch, and the fingers can finely differentiate the nature of stimuli, which the arm or trunk cannot. We use finger tips, not our elbows or knees, to feel an object and identify its characteristics!

Questions were welling up in my mind. What happens to

the brain representation when you amputate one hand? Does it retain its cortical representation, or does the brain use that 'redundant' part of the cortex to do something else?

Answers to these questions may be key to understanding the occurrence of the phantom. From animal studies, we have known for a long time that the representation in the brain can change if the input changes. Merzenich and colleagues from the University of California at San Francisco[10] showed in the 1980s that if you amputate the middle finger of an adult monkey, within two months the area of the brain that normally responds to this digit begins to respond to stimuli delivered to the adjacent fingers. The cortex is therefore flexible or plastic in this regard. These authors also showed that excessive use of a finger by a monkey leads to an expansion of the cortical region devoted to that finger. It was initially thought that this 'expansion' of the region of representation did not extend beyond 1 mm of the cortex, probably because the nerve fibres typically do not branch out to more than 1 mm in the adult brain. Researchers from the National Institute of Health in the United States showed that this view may be incorrect,[11] and cortical reorganisation may occur at much larger distances, perhaps up to a centimetre. On the basis of their study of patients with phantom limbs, Ramachandran and his colleagues showed that the human brain is astonishingly plastic in this regard and reorganises itself rather quickly.[12] The hand area of the cortex, now not receiving input from the amputated hand, is invaded by the face area from one side and the arm area from the other. This suggests that the brain is a dynamic organ that is constantly responding to the input it receives. A consequence of this reorganisation is that there is often a map of the lost hand on the face and the arm stump. In other words, stimulation of parts of the cheek on the same side of the stump evokes sensations in the phantom limb. The brain is tricked into believing that the sensations are coming from the hand that existed previously. Not surprisingly, one theory to explain pain in the phantom limb is that irritation of the nerves in the stump produces a sensation of pain in the phantom. I tried to explain this to Julian as simply as I could.

Julian was happy to accept this explanation of his experience, removing any doubts that might have lingered about his sanity. But he was puzzled about some aspects of the explanation. He was thinking of people born without one or more limbs. Could that person still experience a phantom limb? If the body schema of the brain resides in the genes, this should indeed be the case.

Until the 1960s people believed that children born with missing limbs did not experience phantoms. In 1964 a group of investigators described 13 cases with congenitally missing limbs that developed phantom limbs.[13] Dr Ramachandran reported a case of a 20-year-old woman whose arms were missing from birth and who had a vivid experience of phantom limbs. This suggests that our body schema may be innate. However, our experience does influence the phantom. A person who had a deformed and painful limb before the amputation is likely to experience a phantom with a similar deformity and possibly pain. This brings us to the question of loss of other body parts. What happens if you lose a leg or a nose or an ear or some other appendage? Is there a phantom for these body parts as well?

Our experience of our body shape is of course much more

extensive than just the upper limbs. We generally talk about phantom limbs, and what applies to the arm and hand applies equally well to the leg and foot. This does not mean that the experience is restricted to the limbs. First of all, one does not have to lose a limb to experience the phantom. Patients with injury to the brachial plexus, the bundle of nerves that lies in the armpit and innervates the upper limb, often develop a phantom arm – a kind of third arm – that hangs to the side or is in front of the chest. Blocking the brachial plexus nerves with an anaesthetic will produce this sensation in about 95 per cent of cases.[14] Cases have been described of phantom penises in individuals who underwent amputation of the penis. The phantom penis is reported to even experience erections and ejaculation.[15] After breast removal, about 25 per cent of women have been reported to experience a phantom breast, with the nipple often being the most vivid part. Pain may be experienced in the phantom breast. Phantom of the nose has been described, but I am not aware of any case of a phantom ear. To some extent, the experience of a phantom of another body part will depend upon how vivid the experience of the organ was before the amputation. If it was a painful and gangrenous ear, say after frostbite, it is possible that a phantom will appear. It is interesting that even internal organs can produce phantom experiences. A patient was described whose colon and rectum – parts of the large bowel – were removed, yet he continued to have experiences of bowel movement and flatus. Some women continue to report menstrual cramps after their uterus has been removed. Patients who have had bladder removal owing to cancer sometimes report sensations of a full bladder, and even the experience that they were urinating.

I was beginning to strain Julian's credulity. The only 'phantom' he had heard of previously was the character in the comic books – the ghost who walks. He had never heard of phantom pregnancy, a well-recognised condition, but with a basis different from the phantom limb or similar phenomena we had been discussing.

Phantom pregnancy is in fact a false pregnancy wherein a woman develops all the signs of pregnancy,[16] including swelling of the abdomen, the stopping of the periods, morning sickness, swelling of the breasts and weight gain – she actually believes that she is pregnant. In some cases, she may actually go on to delivery, with of course nothing to deliver. The signs can be so convincing that medical professionals may be fooled until a blood test or an ultrasound examination is done. It is generally thought to be a psychiatric condition, although the psychological basis is not always self-evident. It is of course not related to loss of a body part. On the contrary, it is usually based on a strong desire on the part of the woman to become pregnant. Mary Tudor, Queen of England in the sixteenth century, is said to have had many false pregnancies, ending each time in violent disappointment. In humans therefore, phantom pregnancies probably represent a temporary wish fulfilment. In some animals, false pregnancies may serve a practical purpose. For example, Dalmations and Labradors develop pseudo-pregnancies and begin to lactate, and are therefore able to feed young pups.

We have drifted somewhat from Julian's main problem: the pain in his phantom. Julian told me reluctantly that the hand not only had a presence, it also had life. It would jerk and move, usually involuntarily, but sometimes when he attempted to gesture using both limbs. At other times, it was stiff and immobile, and he could not move it, try as he might. 'If only I could move it!' he mused. 'It would take this awful stiffness and soreness away. It is strange that it moves when I yawn or spread both my hands, yet it is not under my control. The worst part is that the fist is closed tightly, and the nails dig into my palm.' A case of phantom nails digging mercilessly into phantom flesh, I thought to myself. I tried to explain to Julian the possible reasons for his experience of movement, yet a lack of control. Julian's arm was paralysed and painful before the amputation, and it is not unusual for this state to persist in the phantom. Ramachandran called it 'learned paralysis'.[17]

Why was the phantom limb stiff and not under voluntary control? One can only speculate on the possible causes. Julian's limb was immobile after the accident and before the amputation. Is it possible this left a neural signature of some sort such that the limb was paralysed? Normally, when we move an arm, we generate messages in the frontal lobes on the other side of the body in brain regions called the supplementary motor area (SMA), which then directs the motor cortex to send messages to the muscles responsible for the movement. The moving arm provides feedback, visually as well as through sensory, muscle and joint receptors, to tell the brain that the arm has indeed moved. This feedback goes to the parietal lobes of the brain, which also receives input about the motor command sent to the muscles, thus enabling it to integrate the motor and sensory data. In the case of amputation, the motor cortex is still able to send signals down to the muscles, which are no longer present, but the motor part of the brain is possibly not aware of this loss. The lack of feedback information may be responsible for the sense of 'paralysis' that is experienced. This situation can persist even after the limb has been amputated, and may explain why a phantom limb can be paralysed, strange as it may seem. Yet Julian's limb had involuntary movements, and moved during certain actions that involved both upper limbs such as yawning. This may be because the origin of these involuntary movements is not in the motor cortex but in deeper structures, such as the basal ganglia, that are also involved in movement and are responsible for the genesis of movements that are not under conscious control. These commands to the phantom limb to move therefore bypass the motor cortex and the mechanisms of conscious control.

The spasm in the hand was difficult to explain. It had not existed before the amputation, and had evolved gradually. Even more surprisingly, the nails evoked excruciating pain that was felt in the flesh of the palm. How could this stimulation of phantom receptors lead to a sensation of pain? It makes one wonder about the nature of pain and its genesis. Was it due to the irritation of nerve endings at the stump? Alternatively, was it the sense of spasm in the hand muscles that evoked memories of pain due to the digging of nails into the palm? Was there a memory of the pain that resided in the spinal cord rather than in the brain? Will we ever know?

Ramachandran has argued that the pain may be an adverse consequence of the rewiring in the brain. As mentioned previously, lack of sensory input from the amputated limb leads to a reorganisation of the sensory cortex so that the face area takes over what was previously the hand area. This can be shown by touching the face of a patient with a phantom limb, which provokes a sensation in the limb. The sensation is 'modality specific': touch produces a sensation of touch, hot a sensation of heat and cold similarly a sensation of cold. If for some reason cross-wiring occurs in this reorganisation, pain may result from even a soft touch.

After I had seen Julian on two occasions, I had convinced myself that there were no 'psychiatric' causes of his pain. His depression was in fact a response to the pain. Julian's problem was more than just pain; he had stiffness, spasm and a lack of motor control of his phantom limb. How could it be restored to him? I tried to replicate an ingenuous experiment reported by Ramachandran and his colleagues.[18]

'This may sound strange, but we have to try to get you moving your phantom limb,' I said to Julian.

'That would be marvellous – it would be such a relief if this stiffness of the limb could go away,' he replied. He obviously welcomed the idea; also, it was the first time anyone had treated his experiences as reality, and referred to the phantom as if it had a material existence. He now had a partner in his quest.

With the help of a colleague, I had created a 'virtual reality box' along the lines suggested by Dr Ramachandran.[19] This was a cardboard box with the lid removed and a mirror on one of the walls. The front of the box had two holes for Julian to insert his hands – the real hand and the phantom one. When he inserted his left hand into the box, he could see its mirror image where the phantom should have been. I showed him the box and explained the procedure.

'I would like you to try to insert your left hand in this hole and the phantom in the other hole. Now I would like you to make clenching and unclenching movements with both hands as if one is the mirror image of the other.'

Julian was hesitant, but went along with the experiment. His response was ecstatic: 'It moves! Yes, I can move it!'

'Keep doing it,' I responded.

'For the first time I can see the cramp going away. What a relief!'

'Now can you close your eyes and continue to do the movements,' I instructed.

He closed his eyes, and the expression on his face changed. 'It's frozen again. I cannot move it.' There was imploring in his voice.

I asked him to open his eyes again, and his ability to move the hand returned. I asked him to move his hand at the wrist in upward, downward and circular movements. After he had done this for about five minutes, the session was stopped, and he took his 'hands' out of the box. The feeling of stiffness and pain returned.

I explained to him that it would take many sessions before he could expect to get relief. He took the box home, promising to 'practise' the movements many times a day. He rang me two days later, quite excited. 'It stays! The effect stays for many hours. I am beginning to have hope.' I arranged to see him in a week's time and encouraged him to keep practising.

At the time of his visit, he seemed quite pleased with the progress. He could easily unclench his fist and move his wrist with the box, and the effect persisted for many hours after that. The spasm and the 'digging' feeling were greatly relieved. He still felt 'pins and needles' in his phantom hand, but even that feeling was easing. He had gone to visit his friends for the weekend and had taken the box with him. I arranged to see him again in two weeks time. About two weeks later he rang me. 'It's gone! The hand's gone!' he remarked.

'Gone? You mean you no longer have the phantom limb?'

'It's still there but only a few fingers dangling from the stump. The full length of the arm is gone. It happened rather suddenly when I was using the box today.'

'Can you move the fingers?'

'Yes, and the pain and the tingling are not there.'

'Is that a good result?' I asked him.

'I am not quite sure. It probably is a good result. It is something I have been wishing for, but now that it has happened, I am feeling uncertain. In a way, I miss my arm.'

I explained to him the phenomenon of 'telescoping' of the phantom hand, which had previously been described in other patients. He was relieved to know that his was not a unique experience.

Julian had demonstrated an extraordinary capacity of the brain to interact with the environment. On the one hand, the body image has an innate quality about it, suggesting a code we are born with. On the other hand, the brain depends upon visual feedback to complete the picture without which it becomes hopelessly caught in its stable percept. The mirror provided the brain with an image of the hand that it believed existed but which was no longer present. The brain was then able to re-establish control over the hand and move it at will. The percept of the hand could thereby be altered, with the benefit that the pain was no longer present. It makes us see the brain in a fresh light – a flexible machine that modifies itself depending upon the input it receives.

While the brain has a 'structure' of the body stored in it, it weighs any information that comes in before reaching a final decision. When the information reaching the brain from different sources is discrepant, it tries its best to form a coherent picture. In other words, it imposes a reality. The ancient mystics realised this when they referred to the world as a veil or an illusion created by the human mind.[20] Neuroscience, however, would consider the brain as a reality machine that creates reality so as to improve the survival of the individual and the species. Sometimes this reality needs a little nudge.

Julian no longer suffered the pain and distress from his phantom limb. I saw him three months later. His depression had improved, as had his *joie de vivre*. It is strange that he still sometimes missed his phantom. He had come to regard the phantom as something that had tried to keep him 'whole'. Now that he had learnt to feel whole without a limb, the help of the phantom was no longer needed. I reminded him of the dying words of Lord Nelson as he fell on the deck of *Victory* in the final hours of the Battle of Trafalgar, described by the King of England as the most splendid and decisive naval victory: 'Thank God I have done my duty.' Julian's phantom had also done its duty by keeping him whole until he was reconciled to his loss!

10

Freudian slips and semantic slides

Someone said that God gave us memory so that
we might have roses in December.

J. M. Barrie (1860–1937), rectorial address at St Andrew's,
3 May 1922

'Do you think I might be developing dementia?' I have encountered this question in many different settings. At dinner parties, the parents of my friends sometimes struggle with names and dates, and as soon as they find out that I am a neuropsychiatrist, out pops the question. I remember a lecture I gave to the physicians at my hospital. While the topic of the lecture was 'brain stimulation', the first question asked at the end of the lecture – indeed by the elderly chairman himself – was: 'Dr Sachdev, what do you make of the little memory lapses that I and many of my friends seem to suffer from?' I gave some uninformative response at that time. But when Brent confronted me with the same question in the Memory Clinic, I could no longer duck for cover.

Brent was a 70-year-old sprightly man who had always been at the top of his game. He had served as the head of many corporations. Finally, at the age of 55 years, he decided to start his own business, and within five years he had built a very successful enterprise with more than 50 employees. What was the reason for his success?

'I was always full of positive energy, and I could take my employees along with me. I was an effective organiser and worked very well in meetings. You know, much of my success was due to my memory – I never forgot a face and could always place a name next to it. That is, until recently – which is the reason I am here to see you.'

'Please tell me about your problem,' I encouraged him.

'I cannot tell you when it began. I think it has crept upon me – just like the greying of my hair, or the wrinkles on my skin. You look back at the photos of 20 years ago, and it comes as a shock that you have aged. With the mind, you cannot see it that clearly. It probably began a few years ago. I remember a meeting about ten years ago – I can still see that table vividly in my mind's eye. I was speaking and needed to say something to the general manager of my company, sitting to my right. But I could not remember his name. You see, I had known this guy for years, and saw him on a daily basis. It somehow wouldn't come. I knew it was there, in some recess of my brain, but I could not bring it out.'

'Like being on the tip of the tongue,' I prompted.

'Exactly, on the tip of my tongue! If someone had called out his name, I would immediately have known. I was hoping someone would prompt me. Mind you, I covered myself well and did not give it away. I could refer to him in the third person, rather jokingly. I know it was not the first time that I had had difficulty remembering a name, but this one was dramatic as it happened in relation to a colleague I knew so well.'

Brent went on to tell me that this had been happening for

many years. Recently, the lapses have become more frequent. It used to be the occasional name that he forgot. The name would then come back after a few minutes when he was not focusing on it. Nowadays this could happen in a lot of situations, to the point of embarrassment. He had resorted to a generic 'mate' rather than risk addressing his friends by the wrong name. When told someone's name for the first time, he made an extra effort to remember it. If it was important to remember, he took the first opportunity to write it down. He added that he did not generally have difficulties in remembering his family members' names, even when it came to his grandchildren. He might sometimes get stuck – the tip of the tongue again – and had to resort to 'son' or daughter' until he could catch his mental breath again. He was keen to find out if this tip-of-the-tongue 'thing' was a really bad sign.

I was tempted to reassure him. The tip-of-the-tongue experience in itself is quite normal.[1] All of us can recall such instances. The feeling is that the word is there somewhere in the brain, but you just cannot access it. It is therefore associated with a feeling of knowing. I can recall many instances in which it has happened to me. The feeling of knowing is quite strong – as if it will jump out any moment, but the more you try, the worse it gets.

Perhaps it is best understood as a problem of retrieval of information already stored in the memory. Like a good filing system, there are many facets to good memory. You memorise some information, file it in some part of the brain, then retrieve that file when you need it. In tip-of-the-tongue, you know the file is there. You also recognise the nature of the file. You may not remember the name Joan, but you can describe the colour of her eyes, her height, the qualities of her smile – you can recognise her voice. You will find that this biographical information is easier to recall than the name itself. You may even remember the first letter of her name, and you know it is not Jill or Janine or Jacqui. You know the lexical properties of the word, but still cannot get the word out when you want it. Later that day, when you are relaxing in your room, the name suddenly comes to your mind, and you berate yourself for being such an idiot.

Another quality of this phenomenon is that the harder you try, the more futile it seems. Recall of information is normally an automatic process. If it fails, we make a mental effort to search for the information in our mental stores. We first concentrate on the task, which is like shining a mental torch on the landscape we wish to illuminate.[2] This will of course inhibit some other activities the brain is engaged in. We then activate a few strategies to resolve the problem. In the example of Joan, I might try to remember where I last saw her, who else knows her, the clothes she wears, etc, then go through various names letter by letter until one name seems right. The problem with this conscious mental effort is that it suspends some of the automatic processes that have worked in the past. The effortful strategy keeps throwing up an alternative word that in some way blocks the correct word from being brought into consciousness. The psychologist D. M. Burke called it the 'persistent alternate'.[3] At a later time, when you are no longer engaged in this mental effort, the automatic process comes into play successfully and … *voilà*!

There is an interesting twist to this. What happens to deaf-mute individuals who use sign-language? Do they experience

anything akin to a tip-of-the-tongue? Remarkably, yes —
they are known to have what is best called the tip-of-the-
fingers, somewhat ironically. When something is on the tip of
the fingers of a signer, he or she knows the sign but cannot
retrieve it. A few years ago, some researchers at the University of California in San Diego examined 33 deaf signers, all
young adults, and found a number of incidents of this experience, most commonly for proper names.[4] All participants
reported being familiar with the phenomenon, as they had
experienced it at some time in the past. They were asked to
sign the names of famous people such as Audrey Hepburn and
Mikhail Gorbachev whose pictures were presented to them.
When unable to retrieve the name, the signers were able to
recall detailed information about the famous person. They
often reported partial recall of the target sign involving the
hand shape, location and orientation. They also often recalled
the first letter of the name. The authors had given a new meaning to the expression 'on the tip of my fingers'!

What is intriguing about the tip-of-the-tongue phenomenon is the feeling of knowing the name. How does the mind
know that it knows when it cannot tell what it knows? To
some extent that is a mystery. There is certainly a mechanism
in the brain that generates a feeling of knowing. When we are
asked a question, we are aware whether we know the answer or
not. The brain is monitoring the process of retrieval of information, and is aware whether the correct retrieval has occurred
or not. It has looked at alternative answers, and hones in on
the correct answer. This is usually referred to as 'metacogni-
tion', something that supervises the cognitive processes. It is
likely that this is associated with a certain emotional state —

that is why we refer to it as a 'feeling'. The extent to which the emotional brain is activated will determine how strong this feeling is. It is similar to the feeling of knowing that you get when you meet somebody familiar in the street but cannot name the person. The brain somehow signals recognition.

Is it correct to call it a 'feeling' of recognition? Is it not cold, rational thinking? The experience that 'yes, this is right' must have an emotion associated with it. Such evaluations are rarely without emotion. In fact, as the neurologist Antonio Damasio and others have argued,[5] if a person's emotional brain is dissociated from the thinking brain, such judgments become impaired. It is therefore quite appropriate to say that it is indeed a 'feeling' of knowing. There is often a feeling of not knowing, and of course the feeling of knowing can sometimes be wrong – as when you make an error. It is important that you recognise the error, especially if someone points it out to you.

Brent was reassured that tip-of-the-tongue is commonplace and quite normal. He had also noted that it happened a lot more now than it did when he was younger. Should it be regarded just as part of ageing? To some extent that is correct. Older people are slower in recalling names, make more errors and experience more tip-of-the-tongue incidents. If you give people pictures of famous people and ask them to name them, older individuals are more likely to report tip-of-the-tongue experiences. They are also less likely to pick up on a phonological cue, such as 'the name starts with N … Nicole Kidman, of course'. We do not know why this happens. There are some changes in the brain with age that might account for it: the younger brain processes information much more quickly and therefore takes less time to retrieve stored information. It used to be believed that the brain loses nerve cells as it ages. The joke was that after you turned 30, it was all downhill – you lost several thousand nerve cells every day until you could no longer compensate for the losses. We now know that this is not true – neurons do not decrease significantly in number with age. However, their connectedness becomes less efficient – they are no longer as robustly connected with their near and distant neighbours. Since the brain is after all an assembly of networks, the information flow through these networks becomes less efficient with age. This may be the biological basis of some of the inefficiencies of the memory system of older people. But there were other possible explanations as well.

It may also be that with age, there is an overload of information. For retrieving a word from the memory store, we need one or more cues that are linked to the word. The cues to Joan may be her height, the colour of her hair, her occupation, her close friends, the place she last met you, or other such associations. It is more likely that the older person has the same cues linked to many other names – with years of such associations overloading the system, so to speak. The efficiency of the retrieval system is therefore reduced as it is more likely to come up with an alternative name. The semantic tree in the older brain has many more branches – a veritable forest in many ways, making it difficult to negotiate your way. Some of the branches are thick and stand out – you have no difficulty recalling your wife's name, or the name of your dog. This is because the associations with this word have been rehearsed so often that the automaticity does not break down, even when the brain is in a suboptimal state. Imagine yourself totally drunk, or having just woken up from sleep – you will still remember your wife's name without difficulty.

'I would hate to think of the alternative,' Brent chuckled. He had been listening to me carefully. His central concern had, however, not been allayed. 'Let me raise with you again my biggest concern: could these lapses mean that I am going to develop dementia soon?'

I had anticipated this question from him – this was a concern he shared with millions of others who are looking for the red flag of Alzheimer's disease. I had to answer this carefully so as not to be misinterpreted. It is true that early dementia is the harbinger of an increase in such memory lapses. How does one then distinguish between what is routine from the sinister? I often rely on a qualitative change. Individuals with early dementia get less benefit from phonological cues – the name starts with 'He' for 'Hermann'. Their memory stores become extremely difficult to navigate, and the information is often not accessible, even when prompts are available. Not only are they not able to access the name in their stores, they also recall less biographical information associated with particular names or faces. The richness of the stores is depleted, and more recent information is lost in the early stages. In putting names to faces, they are more likely to have difficulty with famous faces from more recent times – they could tell you more about Marilyn Monroe than Princess Diana. This temporal gradient belies common sense. I have met many family members of patients with early dementia who are quite convinced that the patient's memory is good because she can recall information from the past 'much better than they can'. The brain regions preferentially affected by Alzheimer's disease, the most common cause of dementia, are the regions important for remembering new information. They have more difficulty forming new or recent memories rather than very old ones.

Brent seemed to be reassured by my explanation. His pattern of memory difficulties did not seem sinister by this definition. 'I am not therefore at risk of calling my wife Paris or Madonna!' he joked. Yet I was not going to let him get away so easily. Unfortunately, while his memory lapses did not appear to go beyond the ordinary, this distinction was not very precise when it came to diagnosis, and I rely on some standard neuro-psychological tests. Before I did this, I wanted to tell him that his lapses were not Freudian. He said that he often confused his daughters' names, especially if he was angry and had not had time to deliberate on the names. He even remembered an instance in which he called the dog by his daughter's name. What would Dr Freud have said about that?

Sigmund Freud, the father of psychoanalysis, did state in his earlier work that there was always an unconscious wish or a desire that lay beneath such mistakes. The unconscious wish, however, played out a childhood conflict in most cases. The joke is that 'in an ordinary slip, you say one thing and mean another, but in a Freudian slip, you say one thing and mean your mother'. His book *Psychopathology of Everyday Life* makes interesting reading, but I think that some of the concepts, including the one on 'Freudian slips', have been vulgarised. Sigmund Freud argued that forgetting or a false recall of a name was often due to suppression of the name because of its association with a repressed desire or motivation, usually linked to a sexual or hostile impulse. The fact that the real desire was repressed meant that the basis of the slip was not transparent. A psychoanalytical exploration was necessary to unravel the unconscious motivation. Depending upon what he found upon his exploration, Dr Freud would not be kind in his interpretation if you called your wife by your daughter's name, or by another woman's name. He might be more forgiving if you mistook one daughter for another.

To quote from Freud:

> I was led to examine exhaustively the phenomenon of temporary forgetfulness through the observation of certain peculiarities, which, although not general, can, nevertheless, be seen clearly in some cases. In these there is not only forgetfulness, but also false recollection: he who strives for the escaped name brings to consciousness others – substitutive names – which, although immediately recognized as false, nevertheless obtrude themselves with great tenacity. The process which should lead to the reproduction of the lost name is, as it were, displaced, and thus brings one to an incorrect substitute.
>
> Now it is my assumption that the displacement is not left to psychic arbitrariness, but that it follows lawful and rational paths. In other words, I assume that the substitutive name (or names) stands in direct relation to the lost name, and I hope, if I succeed in demonstrating this connection, to throw light on the origin of the forgetting of names.[6]

Brent confessed to all sorts of slips. 'I have sometimes called my golf buddies by the wrong names, only to correct myself immediately after. I said only the other day that the Roosters had won, when I meant they had lost. I called gerberas chrysanthemums – would you believe it? I am sure Dr Freud would have a field day if you let him loose on me.'

I told him that amateur psychologists have had a field day at the expense of Freud. Even Sigmund Freud admitted that not all forgetfulness or slips – 'parapraxes', as they are sometimes called – are due to repressed wishes of sexual or violent nature. There might be much simpler explanations. I like to call them 'semantic slides'. When you go out to retrieve a word, you slide on to something else that is a neighbour. The technical term would be 'lexical retrieval errors'. Brent had noticed that when he mistook his daughter's name, it was usually with his other daughter. A friend's name is replaced with another friend, a flower with another flower. Your mental searchlight has brought you to the correct region in the brain, only to let you down at the final step. And, again as Brent had identified, it did not happen only with people's names – the names of common objects were also affected.

And there isn't always a sexual motivation! Some people believe that if it has a whiff of sexuality, it must somehow be Freudian. There is the apocryphal story of a medical student who was examining the chest of a buxom lady. As part of the auscultation process, it is usual to ask the patient to take big or deep breaths. His rather embarrassing slip was his entreaty for 'big breasts'. Then there is the story of the newspaper article on the soldier who had been through many a battle that referred to him as *bottle*-scarred, only to publish an apology the following day to this *battle*-scared soldier. Freudian interpretations, irrespective of whether or not you believed in his methods, do not lie so much on the surface.

Brent liked the simpler non-Freudian explanation of a semantic slide. After all, the brain is not a computer that comes up with exactly the right word every time. Slips must have something to do with how the brain stores words and how it is able to retrieve them from the storage. If it was a simple matter of filing words in discrete compartments, like books in a library, the retrieval system would either succeed or fail – there would not be near misses with help from semantic[7] and phonological cueing. The computer uses a binary code and very simple logical rules for its storage. No wonder there are no near-misses and slips-of-the-LCD. The brain is not silicon hardware – it is a soggy mush of billions of cells that are massively interconnected, and it is living and breathing and changing all the time. It is a miracle therefore that it can be as predictable in its reactions as it normally is. The fact that it has semantic slides and near misses must tell us about the way language is stored in the brain – indeed it might reveal the brain basis of knowledge in general. Of course, the brain – and by inference the mind – does not reveal its secrets all at once. We must nibble away at the little cues so that rays of light will penetrate.

One method to decipher these secrets has been to study the evolution of language. Animals do have methods of communication and, when it comes to the primates, rudimentary aspects of language are already in existence. Charles Darwin wrote about the rich repertoire of symbolic communication between animals, but linguists do not classify such forms of communication as language. The human brain evolved language from these symbols. Dolphins are said to call each other by names,[8] much like humans, but are not known to use language for other communication. Apes in captivity have been taught to sign, and some like Kanzi[9] were able to be taught several hundred words. One can argue that the larynx and the speech apparatus of apes preclude the development of human-like sounds. Vervet monkeys have been studied in the wild to produce a variety of sounds with different meanings, such as the 'snake call' and the 'eagle call', which other monkeys appear to understand. The animal communication lacks syntax and grammar, and therefore cannot be called even proto-language.[10] It can be argued that the complexity of human neocortex was necessary for language to develop.[11]

It has been suggested that humans come to the world already with a brain primed to acquire language – that the child has an innate ability to acquire the grammar and syntax of any language. It is interesting that all human beings have the ability to use language to a similar extent. They can translate, borrow or invent words to express all the relevant concepts, which is remarkable considering that some groups, such as the Tasmanian Aborigines, were isolated from the rest of the world for more than 40 000 years. If you take a newborn child from any part of the world and place it in another part, it has no difficulty in acquiring the local language to the same extent as the locals. The brain does not seem to favour one language over another, at least in the first year of life.

My musings had digressed from what I had begun with: Brent's memory lapses involved proper nouns, but were beginning to affect other aspects of his language, including common nouns and verbs. But many fascinating questions remained. Let's take the case of proper names. Why is it that when you lose memory, you experience the greatest difficulty with proper names rather than other words? It may well have to do with the nature of these words. Proper nouns are unusual in that they have a purely referent function: they refer to a particular person or object but not to any properties or attributes. The link between people and their names is arbitrary, often based on the baptismal act, but it acquires certain rigidity in relation to its designation. This rigidity might mean that the brain has a limited number of neural connections dealing with a name, reducing the redundancy and making it more vulnerable to any disruption. A highly redundant system will have multiple associations and, therefore, many possibilities for the information to be retrieved. When the referent is so specific, any change in the brain, be it related to ageing or neurodegeneration as in dementia, is likely to disrupt the function. The retrieval process is also more likely to be blocked by another name with a stronger association.

Many of my patients have told me that the greatest difficulty is with names of people. Even other proper nouns, such as names of capitals of countries, are sometimes difficult to remember. There is no difficulty with names of common objects, but as the objects become uncommon or more specific, the old brain begins to groan. Brent gave an instructive example.

'Spotting flowers used to be my favourite pastime, but flower shops now provoke much anxiety. My wife loves gerbera bouquets with their varied colours, and I must have bought hundreds in my lifetime. There I was in the shop the other day, and the word "gerbera" escaped me altogether. I had to disguise my lapse by using pronouns and pointing to the flowers. I consoled myself in a Shakespearean way by saying that my wife will still love them much the same even if I could not name them.'

This was revealing about the way in which the brain stores information. There is a particular referent – the gerbera – a special kind of flower that Brent wished to name. The word flower is also a referent, but for a particular class of objects. The brain stores information about both the common and the particular, and the two are intimately connected. Retrieval of the common is certainly easier. It is hard to imagine a person being able to recall the name 'gerbera' and not being able to say it was a flower. The reverse is often not true – you can say it is a flower, but not what kind of flower. The word 'flower' also evokes a certain flow of associations that define its common characteristics – all flowers occur on plants, have petals of various colours, are involved in the reproductive cycle of the plant, and so forth. Many flowers have a characteristic scent that can evoke a memory without seeing the flower. Flowers may have other associations: the first love that was consummated with a dozen red roses or white lilies that covered the coffin of a dear friend. The emotional memory they evoke can be intense.

One must marvel at the various associations that a common word can elicit. Even more marvellous is that these associations must involve quite different brain regions, suggesting a network that operates efficiently and at very high speed. The memory of a scent is stored differently by the brain as opposed to a memory of colour, or the memory of the beloved who was the recipient of the roses. Yet these memories have a common theme of 'flower'. The stuff that birds and bees do is also intimately linked to the concept of flower. For an Australian digger a red poppy might commemorate a fallen soldier at Gallipoli. A

Chinese herbalist sees in flowers the cure of all ailments imaginable. Flowers are therefore also linked to abstract concepts, which the brain must necessarily deal with differently.

This brings us to the age-old questions: is it true that all knowledge is linked to all other knowledge in the brain? This is the question that has occupied the creative energies of many neuropsychologists: how does the brain store knowledge, and how is it that we can access vast amounts of knowledge in an instant, and often with uncritical certainty? Our understanding of this has been put together piece by tiny piece. There are some natural experiments that have shed light in unusually dark corners.

Investigators from Italy reported the case of GC, a 59-year old woman who gradually lost the ability to remember proper names.[12] She spoke normally during a conversation, with no word-finding difficulty or errors in the use of words. She could not, however, name people, including her mother's and daughter's names. She could recall other information about the people she wished to name, such as their telephone numbers and dates of birth, and could even produce the initial letter of the name. To quote the authors: 'She tried to explain the surname Alberti as follows: "Their name starts with A, like the lady writing the horoscopes on magazines, who is an actor's sister, who produces a liqueur starting with S (Strega) in that town with B (Benevento), which is close to the other one with A (Avellino)."' These sentences were produced at a fast rate. Apart from this deficit that she described as a memory deficit ('I have lost my memory for names'), she did not show any other apparent language impairment.'[13]

The investigators gave her a number of tests. She was of

normal intelligence and could attend to tasks and retain information in her mind at an average level. She could remember lists of words normally, and her understanding of language was also normal. She was able to detect the name of famous people from a list that intermingled famous with non-famous names, scoring 47 out of 50. She was able to state whether the person was an actor, a politician or a sportsperson. She was able to name common objects and body parts, but had difficulty naming musical instruments. Her major difficulty was in coming up with proper nouns, either when she was given a letter to produce the names or shown pictures or verbal descriptions of famous people. She could name colours and cars. When given the descriptions of 25 famous Italians, she was able to name only four. Interestingly, she was able to come up with the first letter of the name, or choose between three alternative letters in about a third of the cases.

Brain scans of this patient showed atrophy or loss of brain tissue in the left temporal lobe, with a decreasing gradient from the front to the back. Blood flow to this brain region was also reduced, suggesting that it was functioning at a suboptimal level. She was suffering from a lobar atrophy or reduction in size of parts of the brain, which was possibly the early stage of a fronto-temporal dementia.[14] It is interesting to speculate whether this and other similar cases suggest a neural basis for proper nouns, as if this knowledge is located in a specific brain region. Both temporal lobes have been suggested to be involved in person-related information. Abnormalities of the left temporal lobe have generally been linked with names of people, whereas the right temporal lobe has been associated with faces. Patients with loss in the right temporal lobe tend to lose information that refers to themselves, that which has a strong emotional component and some autobiographical information.

Investigators from the University of Cambridge described a patient, VH, who suffered right temporal lobe atrophy (loss of nerve cells) initially.[15] He had severe difficulty identifying people from their faces, but did better with names and voices. Although he had always lived in England, he was unable to recognise a photograph of Margaret Thatcher, and could not provide any information about her when presented with the name. As his disorder worsened and his left temporal lobe became more affected, his semantic deficits became more prevalent. The brain does have some degree of anatomical specialisation of semantic knowledge, although nature does hold surprises for us. It seems that when it comes to person-related information, both temporal lobes are important, and if the damage is greater to the left side, naming becomes affected preferentially.

I was intrigued by the fact that GC could not name musical instruments. Is there a special place in the brain for musical instruments? It raises the question that neuroscientists have agitated over: how is word knowledge stored in the brain? I have already referred to the so-called tree of knowledge. The stem of this tree might be regarded as the distinction between living and non-living objects, with the animate beings further branching into land animals, birds and water animals, and so on. Confusion is more likely to occur with other members populating the same branch. A person with brain damage is more likely to call a hippopotamus a horse than a cat, and certainly not likely to call it an eagle. This may be the reason that when Brent experienced semantic slides, he interchanged his daughters' names, but was unlikely to call them Ivana or Farida, also female names but quite remote from his ethnic group. His daughters' names presumably sat very closely on the same branch of this tree, and a slight error could lead to the mistake. Your dog's name is a special case. While it is an animal, it has a human name and is treated much like your children. It is part of the family, as they say. Its associations for retrieval are therefore likely to be shared with those for your children, and hence the mistaken naming of the dog when you mean your daughter.

This, however, seems to be too simple an explanation, and disregards the fact that the brain is an unbelievably complex network in which knowledge cannot be said to reside safely in one nook. The brain may work as a hierarchy of networks, with each feature being represented in one network and its connections. 'Four legs' may be one such feature that is super-ordinate for dogs and lions and other animals. 'Domesticated vs wild' may be another feature that overlaps the 'four-legged' feature. It is the coming together of a number of such features that determines a category. One can regard these features as fragments of the whole concept, and many fragments must converge for the entity to be revealed. This concept of a series of overlapping networks has been called the 'seman-tic net' theory of knowledge. Since category concepts have common attributes, they are accessed more frequently by the brain, and therefore develop more robust neural representa-tions. They can also be represented by fewer fragments. They are therefore less likely to be disrupted than particular names. For the recall of a particular entity or person, common as well as specific features must be linked, and becomes a slightly more precarious process. An interesting case, FC, was described by McKenna and Warrington,[16] two neuropsychologists from the Institute of Neurology in London. This patient, a sales manager by profession, developed a tumour in his left temporal lobe, which affected his ability to produce names. When shown a picture of Mahatma Gandhi, he said 'India', suggesting that the recognition and some associations were preserved but that the proper name was not accessible.

There is some evidence that the brain deals with different categories differently. Let's take the case of living and non-living things. This was recognised as early as 1946 when Johannes Nielsen described a patient who had more difficulty identifying inanimate objects by sight or touch than living things.[17] He could identify foods only by their taste. Nielsen later described a patient who showed the reverse pattern, arguing that a specific brain region had been responsible for this dissociation. Some interesting cases demonstrating this were described by Dr Elizabeth Warrington and her colleagues in London.[18] They had two patients, JBR and SBY, who had suffered from a brain infection with herpes simplex, a virus that tends to affect the temporal lobes of the brain in particular. When shown pictures of inanimate objects, they were able to achieve a 70–80 per cent success in identifying the object, and a greater than 50 per cent success in naming it. When shown foods, their success rate dropped to 20–25 per cent. However, when shown pictures of living things, the success in identifying or naming was only 6–7 per cent. How might this be? One suggestion is that we associate living things with function, whereas inanimate objects are more often associated with sensory phenomenon. Let's take an example.

When patients with abnormality in the temporal lobe are asked to describe a dog, they typically say 'they bark', or 'they are your friends' or 'you feed them', and not their shape, size or colour. A soccer ball, on the other hand, is likely to be described as 'it's round, usually black and white', etc. This may be an over-simplification, however, as the ball also 'bounces' and 'is used to play the most popular game in the world'.

Brent was familiar with the recent case of the little girl who had been abandoned by her father and had been nicknamed Pumpkin by the police and the Australian media. It is not difficult to believe that vegetables are remembered differently from humans. Antonio Damasio and colleagues described a patient, AN, who could name only 50 per cent of the stimuli shown, but he could provide some description of all the objects, suggesting that he could recognise them. When shown animals or vegetables, his success at naming them were 38 per cent and 19 per cent respectively. With human faces, his performance was down to 10 per cent. When shown tools, however, his performance jumped to 70 per cent. The distinction between humans and fruits and vegetables can be artificially blurred by some abstract concepts. We often refer to someone as the 'apple of my eye', or as 'cool as a cucumber', 'as red as a beetroot', 'wrinkled as a prune' or 'a tough nut to crack'. The word 'pumpkin' is used as an endearment in the American South and Midwest, although in Japan it refers to an unattractive woman. The abandoned girl in the Australian news was named Pumpkin because of her broad and endearing face.

When used in this manner, 'pumpkin' becomes an abstract word. Is abstract knowledge a different category of knowledge? The brain does seem to deal with abstract words differently from concrete words. This was shown recently in a bilingual patient, IRQ.[19] Concrete words included common nouns (e.g. fruits, body parts, musical instruments) and proper nouns (e.g. famous people, cities), while abstract words denoted concepts (e.g. deceit, trick, steal, cheat). Concrete words appear to lead to more semantically similar errors. For example, 'boat', 'yacht', 'kayak', 'vessel', 'dinghy', 'ferry' and 'ship' are semantically similar words that are in the same category. Abstract words, on the other hand, lead to errors that are semantically associated. An example of this is the list of words 'exercise', 'healthy', 'fitness', 'jogging', 'gymnasium', 'treadmill' etc. It seems that concrete words have a categorical network in the brain whereas abstract words have a semantic network.

Moreover, IRQ was bilingual. What happens when we have two languages stored in the brain? Do they have different compartments? To answer this, we need to understand that there are two aspects to language: the lexicon and the semantics, or, in other words, the dictionary of words and the meanings and concepts entailed. There is controversy on how these are dealt with by the brain in bilingual individuals, with most investigators believing that the lexicons for the two languages have different representations but that the semantics or the concepts are shared. This may explain why the words of a new language may be lost with brain damage or dementia. Many bilingual patients who lose their language ability after a stroke have a differential recovery in their languages – and it is generally their primary language that recovers first.[20] This may be the language that they acquired first or use greatly, or the language spoken in their immediate environment.

Memory disorder researchers at the University of California

in Los Angeles[21] examined patients with early dementia who were bilingual and spoke English as well as another language, most often Spanish. Most of these patients had been regularly exposed to English since the age of about 13 years. In the early stages of dementia, these individuals began to use less English and showed a greater preference for their original language. When speaking English, they were more likely to have intrusions of words and phrases from their mother tongue. It was as if the older neural networks were more resistant to damage by the disease, while the networks acquired later in life were more easily disrupted. We all know that even the lack of usage of a newly learnt language leads to gradual loss of the vocabulary. I brush up my rudimentary French every time I go to France, but it never has a lasting effect.

But the words of the second language are closely associated with those of the first. Bilingual people with early dementia have great difficulty separating their languages. An even more interesting aspect of secondary languages is that when you acquire a third or a fourth language, your semantic errors are likely to occur between your secondary languages. My daughter is a native English speaker but she also speaks Hindi, the most popular Indian language. She has been learning French at school, and when she is speaking French in an excited manner, she sometimes lapses into Hindi without even noticing the transition. It has occasionally left her friends puzzled. On the other hand, when speaking to her grandmother in Hindi, she has occasionally lapsed into French when she is struggling to convey her message in her rudimentary Hindi.

Brent, like most Australians, was completely monolingual. Did it mean that his ageing brain was less likely to be confused? Well, the news on this front may be disappointing for Brent. Researchers in Canada recently showed that being bilingual offered some protection against dementia: dementia first showed up in lifelong bilinguals about four years later than in monolinguals.[22] We have known for some time that children who successfully complete bilingual instruction perform better academically. If their mastery of both languages is at a high level, their performance is even better. They tend to display a certain degree of flexibility in their cognitive functions, and this may be the reason that it has a protective effect against cognitive loss later in life. In fact, many schools may be doing a disservice by keeping their students monolingual. If the government needs another reason to introduce a second language in all primary schools, it is that it may reduce the health bill due to dementia many decades from now.

This has been a long digression. But how was I to decide clinically that Brent was not in the early stages of Alzheimer's?

To form a reliable clinical judgment, I needed to perform a few investigations. I performed a full neurological examination on Brent, and he showed no abnormality. His blood pressure was normal. He had mild diabetes, which was being treated by a specialist. He had been a smoker in the past, but gave it up three decades ago. His cholesterol had also been high in the past and was being treated with a statin (a cholesterol-lowering drug). I requested the clinical neuropsychologist to perform a detailed neuropsychological assessment, and I sent him for a few blood tests and a brain MRI scan. My prediction was that the results of these tests would essentially be normal. After

having spent some time with Brent, I was increasingly confident that he did not have cognitive impairment outside what
was normal for his age.

Unfortunately, age does lead to brain changes. Many older
brains have changes that resemble those seen in Alzheimer's
disease but do not show the full picture of the disorder. It
can be debated whether this is simply very early disease that
will eventually show up in the clinic, but even in the presence
of these changes, the neuronal numbers are not reduced. It
seems that nerve cells do not die with age. What seems more
likely is that their networks become less efficient. Most of
these studies have been conducted in animals – in particular
monkeys and our other primate cousins – and one must be
cautious in applying them to humans. The work does suggest
that the complexity of the neuronal networks is gradually
compromised. A typical neuron has one large fibre called the
axon and a number of smaller branches called dendrites, which
further branch and subbranch into a dendritic tree. These
dendrites link the neuron to other neurons, forming a vastly
complex network. The dendrites carry small protrusions like
mushroom heads that are smaller than a micrometre and can be
seen only by special microscopes. All principal neurons in the
brain carry these spines on their dendrites and, for some nerve
cells, these can number in the tens of thousands. They form
links with spines of other neurons in junctions called synapses
through which information flows from one neuron to another.
The spines are very flexible structures and, using laser scanning
microscopes, it has been shown that they can change over short

periods of time, depending upon the nature of the input into the neuron. It has been shown that with ageing, the dendritic spines become less dense.[23] There are other changes as well, especially in relation to the synapses.

Brent's neuropsychological assessment was normal for his age, although there was evidence that he had most likely slowed down compared to what he would have been in his younger years. His brain scan showed no evidence of shrinkage more than what would be expected at his age. His scan did show scattered abnormalities in the white matter, which are quite common in the elderly, and possibly represent disease of small blood vessels in the brain. Another sign of ageing! He had passed the tests, and the diagnosis was 'a healthy old man'.

What could he do to keep his dendritic spines in prime condition? I discussed with him some of the known modifiable risk factors for dementia. Diabetes was one such factor that needed attention, and he had kept his weight low and was on regular anti-diabetic medication. His blood sugar levels were being regularly monitored. His cholesterol level was normal with the medication he was taking. He had started himself on gingko, a Chinese herb, which I did not advise him to discontinue but did inform him that scientific evidence for its efficacy was lacking. He was also taking vitamin E regularly. Vitamin E is a powerful anti-oxidant, and since there is evidence that oxidation is an important mechanism for ageing as well as dementia, anti-oxidants have had much theoretical support. Unfortunately evidence that it really helps is lacking, as is true for the many other anti-oxidants that people take. The same is true for a range of vitamins. Brent also consumed one or two glasses of red wine with his evening meal, and I supported its continuation. Alcohol has a complex relationship with cognition, with emerging evidence that its consumption in moderation is likely to be good for the brain, but large amounts are clearly harmful. While this may be true of all alcohol, there is some evidence that wine, in particular of the red variety, may have a special protective property because of its content of polyphenols in addition to the ethanol. Alcohol in moderation may also be beneficial for the heart, but its effect on other body organs is not necessarily benign. Because of this, if someone is already drinking regularly, I emphasise the importance of moderation, with no more than two drinks a day, four to five times a week. For someone who does not drink, I do not recommend beginning to do so.

Most importantly, I emphasise the importance of regular physical exercise and mental activity. In my interactions with Brent, I had encountered a mentally very active man. I commended him on this, and encouraged him to continue a range of mental activities. I also emphasised regular physical exercise. He was only too keen to increase his golf to three times a week and make his tennis game weekly. And he promised me that he would walk home from the clinic – a good six kilometres of undulating road. I looked at his shoes – slip-ons best suited to walking on the beach – and suggested that it could wait another day.

Notes

1 The Yipping Tiger

1 Readers new to golf may have difficulties with some of the terms used by golfers. A scratch player is someone with a zero handicap. On a regular 18-hole course, he/she expects to complete the round in 72 strokes or less.

2 Putts are the short strokes with which the golfer hits the ball along the ground to put it in the hole. They require the greatest amount of coordination. They usually require a special club called the putter.

3 Golf has stayed in the Armour family. His grandson Tommy Armour III is a two-time winner on the PGA tour. It is also interesting to point out that golf uses a number of birds' names to describe the number of strokes used to complete one hole: from the 4-under par 'condor' to the 'albatross', 'eagle' and 1-under par 'birdie', to the 2-over par 'hawk', all the way up to the record-breaking 'archaeopteryx'.

4 John Schlee, US Open runner-up in 1973, is reported to have said: 'Watching Sam Snead practice hitting golf balls is like watching a fish practice swimming.' Snead was considered by many to be the best natural player of golf ever.

5 Foster JB. Putting on the agony. World Medicine 1977; 29:26–7.

6 Sachdev PS. Golfer's cramp: Clinical characteristics and evidence against it being an anxiety disorder. Movement Disorders 1992; 4:326–32.

7 McDaniel KD, Cummings JL, Shain S. The 'yips': A focal dystonia of golfers. Neurology 1989; 39:192–5.

8 Lees AJ. *Tics and Related Disorders*. Edinburgh: Churchill Livingston, 1985.

9 Gowers (1845–1915) has been described by some as the greatest clinical neurologist of all time. His *Manual of Diseases of the Nervous System*, first published in 1886 and later dubbed the 'Bible of Neurology' for many years, contains a chapter on writer's cramp that makes interesting reading.

10 Some occupations, such as the shorthand typist, are becoming extinct in

the age of digital recording and word processing. The ranks of writer's cramp victims are therefore shrinking.

2 Shaking hands with Dr Strangelove

1   Singer J. *Androgyny*. Garden City, NY: Anchor Press, 1976, pp222–3. Dr Singer is a Jungian psychoanalyst.

2   For a recent review of the interhemispheric interactions following partial and complete callosotomy, see Funnell M, Corballis PM, Gazzaniga MS. Cortical and subcortical interhemispheric interactions following partial and complete callosotomy, Archives of Neurology, 2000; 57(2):185–9. This review draws our attention to what has been learned about the integrative function of the corpus callosum in the intact brain, and the role of specialisation in hemispheric processing of visual perception, imagery, language, memory and other areas of perception and cognition.

3   Goldstein K. Zur der motorischen Apraxie. J für Psychologie und Neurologie 1908; 11:169–87.

4   Ibid., pp169–70.

5   Akelaitis AI. Studies on corpus callosum. IV. Diagonistic dyspraxia in epileptics following partial and complete section of the corpus callosum. American Journal of Psychiatry 1944–45; 101:594–9.

6   Bundick T Jr, Spinella M. Subjective experience, involuntary movement, and posterior alien hand syndrome. Journal of Neurology, Neurosurgery and Psychiatry 2000; 68(1):83–5.

7   Brion S, Jedynak CP. Trobles du transfert interhemispherique: à propos de trois observations de tumeurs du corps calleux. Le signe de al main étrangère. Revue Neurologique 1972; 126:257–66.

8   Bogen JE. The callosal syndromes. In KM Heilman, E Valenstein (eds). *Clinical Neuropsychology*, 1st edn. New York: Oxford University Press, 1979, pp333–4.

9   Della Sala S, Marchetti C, Spinnler H. Right-sided anarchic (alien) hand: A longitudinal study. Neuropsychologia 1991; 29:1113–27.

10 Geschwind DH, Iacoboni M, Mega MS et al. Alien hand syndrome: Interhemispheric motor disconnection due to a lesion in the midbody of the corpus callosum. Neurology 1995; 45:802–8.

11 Brion S, Jedynak CP. *Les Troubles du Transfert Interhémispherique*. Paris: Masson, 1975.

12 Ambivalence is a psychodynamic concept in which the sufferer is said to harbour opposing emotions (e.g. love and hate) for a person, or contradictory intentions towards an act. The conflict of the two hands evokes the conflicts so dear to psychoanalysis.

13 There are many stories of intermanual conflict in other patients. A particularly interesting one was narrated by Dr Joseph Bogen of the University of Southern California, Los Angeles (in Reeves AG. *Epilepsy and the Corpus Callosum*. New York: Plenum Press, 1984, p518): 'He had been shopping with his wife, something he had not been able to do before the operation. He was sitting next to her in the car as she was driving home. Between them was a large bag of groceries. He recounted, "My left hand reached in the bag and pulled out the licorice she had purchased for herself." I asked him, "Well, what's the matter with that?" He said, "I don't like licorice." I said, "Well, that is strange – what happened?" He said, "I ate it – but I didn't like it."'

14 For an excellent account of hemispheric specialisation, I can recommend the classic text by Sally Springer and Geog Deutsch, *Left Brain, Right Brain*, New York: WH Freeman & Co., 1993.

15 For Myers, consciousness extended not only deeper into the recesses of the brain but also far beyond the physical or terrene world. He was interested in explaining the inexplicable – psychical or paranormal phenomena – and attributed them to 'subliminal uprushes' from the enveloping mother-consciousness into the terrestrial consciousness. William James, the brilliant American psychologist, was impressed by Myers' ideas, which now appear quite bizarre to us.

16 A ouija (pronounced 'weejah') board is a flat board with numbers, letters and a movable 'message board' that helps to spell out messages, which presumably are from supernatural entitites.

17 Myers' theory was severely criticised by Pierre Janet, a contemporary of Freud whose work on hysteria was highly influential.

18 Bourru H, Burot F. Les variations de la personalité. Revue de l'Hypnotisme Expérimental et Thérapeutique 1886–87; 1:193–9, 261–5. This case went on to become one of the most extensively studied cases of male hysteria in the nineteenth century. He was discussed by a string of distinguished physicians, including Ribot, Camuset, Richer, Legrand du Saulle, Jules Voisin and William James. I am indebted to Anne Harrington who drew my attention to this and other nineteenth-century thought on the topic in her excellent book, *Medicine, Mind, and the Double Brain*, Princeton, NJ: Princeton University Press, 1987.

19. Myers FWH. Multiplex personality. Nineteenth Century 1886; 20:648–66.

20. Metals and magnets have been used in medicine since time immemorial. Their prominence in mid-nineteenth-century Europe is attributed to Victor Burq, who 'discovered' that certain metals exerted powerful influences on patients with hysteria. His claims were investigated and

given the thumbs up by a committee of the Société de Biologie in Paris, which included none other than Jean-Martin Charcot.

21 Any parallels with the political right and left are entirely fortuitous.

22 Bruce L. Notes of a case of dual brain action. Brain 1895; 18:54–65.

23 Bleuler E. Halbseitiges Delirium. Psychiatrisch-Neurologische Wochenschrift 1902–03; 4(34):361–7.

24 Janet P. *L'automatisme psychologique*. Paris: Librairie Felix Alcan, 1889, p 414.

25 Liepmann was an associate and admirer of Wernicke. The patient he described was Herr T., who had suffered from a stroke and was diagnosed with 'aphasia and mental disorder'.

26 In clinical neurology, these tasks may be such as make a fist, tap at the door, comb your hair, etc.

27 Liepmann H. Der weitere Kranksheitsverlauf bei dem einseitig Apraktischen und der Gehirnbefund auf Grund von Serienschnitten. Monatsschrift für Psychiatrie und Neurologie 1906; 19(Jan–Jun):217–43.

28 From the Greek *prasso*, meaning 'to do'. He called apraxia 'an aphasia of the extremities'. The argument was that just as a part of the brain was responsible for the orchestration of the intricacies of speech, another part was coordinating the complexity of motor acts. See the case of the Yipping Tiger in chapter 1 for a more detailed discussion.

29 Sperry R. Lateral specialization in the surgically separated hemispheres. In Schmitt F, Worden F (eds). Third Neurosciences Study Program. Cambridge, MA: MIT Press, 1974, 3:5–19.

30 I again refer the reader to *Medicine, Mind, and the Double Brain*, the excellent historical account by Anne Harrington.

31 Libet B, Gleason CA, Wright EW. Time of conscious intention to act in relation to onset of cerebral activity: Readiness potential. Brain 1983; 106:623–42.

32 Gottlieb D, Robb K, Day B. Mirror movements in the alien hand syndrome. Case report. American Journal of Physical Medicine and Rehabilitation 1992; 71:297–300. Their two patients had lesions in the frontal and parietal lobes and not the corpus callosum.

33 This argument has been presented by Dr R Persaud in a letter to the Journal of Neurology, Neurosurgery and Psychiatry 1999; 67(1):130–1.

34 Allen LS, Gorski RA. Sexual orientation and the size of the anterior commissure in the human brain. Proc Natl Acad Sci 1992; 89:7199–202.

3 Swearing like a Spanish sailor

1 'Gilles de la Tourette Syndrome' or 'Tourette's Syndrome' or simply

'Tourette's'. See Stevens H. Syndrome by serendipity. American Journal of Psychiatry 1971; 128:489–92.

2   Tics are the characteristic symptoms of Tourette's and are sudden, rapid, involuntary movements or vocalisations, which are experienced as irresistible, although suppressible for varying periods of time. Common motor tics are eye-blinking, facial grimacing, squinting, head jerking, shoulder shrugging and arm extending. Common vocalisations are throat clearing, grunting, sniffing, barking, snorting, coughing, spitting, humming and screaming. For a detailed exposition of these symptoms, see Shapiro AK, Shapiro ES, Young JG, Feinberg TE. *Gilles de la Tourette Syndrome*. New York: Raven Press 1988, or Comings D. *Tourette Syndrome and Human Behaviour*. Los Angeles, CA: Hope Press 1990.

3   They reportedly occur in about 15 per cent of patients, according to an international multi-site database kept by Dr Freeman in Canada. The results vary from one report to another. The rates are lowest (at about 6 per cent) in Tourette's patients who have a 'pure' disorder, with only tics being present. In those with co-morbid conditions, the rate goes up.

4   Gilles de la Tourette (1857–1904) was a gifted pupil of the famous French neurologist Charcot, and his colourful life is recorded by Guilly (1982) and Lees (1986; see below). In 1884 he described nine patients with '*maladie des tics*', which was named Gilles de la Tourette illness by Charcot. There are some early recorded cases that could possibly be Tourette's. Prince de Conde, a nobleman in the seventeenth-century court of Louis XIV, is noted to have stuffed objects into his mouth to suppress an involuntary bark (Stevens, Syndrome by serendipity – see note 1 above). Another celebrated case is that of Dr Samuel Johnson (1709–84), the towering literary figure in Britain in the eighteenth century (for a detailed discussion of Johnson's movement disorder see: Murray TJ. Dr Samuel Johnson's movement disorders. British Medical Journal 1979; 1:1610–14). However, Johnson was never noted to swear. The first well-documented case of this syndrome is attributable to Itard (1825), who described the famous Marquise de Dampierre with her strange grimaces, contortions, utterances and coprolalia. The cases of the same patient and eight others were together published by Tourette in 1885, leaving his stamp on the disorder. Guilly, a French neuropsychiatrist, describes him rather unflatteringly as 'a scatterbrained, irrational eccentric, or keeping to medical terminology, a hypomaniac on a basis of temperamental lack of balance, ending a short life in a state of dementia'. The more vivid descriptions of Gilles come from Leon Daudet, son of the famous French novelist Alphonse Daudet: 'Gilles de la Tourette was ugly like a

Papuan idol with bundles of hair stuck on it. He was neither good nor bad, neither studious nor lazy, neither intelligent nor foolish, and he vacillated with his confused and malicious mind between a multitude of faults without lingering ...' At the age of 35 he was shot three times by a woman suffering from a paranoid disorder. Gilles might not have been the most brilliant of Charcot's pupils, but he was extremely loyal to the Master. He spent his last years in a clinic in Lausanne, 'very disturbed', and possibly suffering from neurosyphilis. See (for a biographical review) Lees AJ. Georges Gilles de la Tourette: The man and his times. Revue Neurologique (Paris) 1986; 142:808–16; Itard JMG. Mémoire sur quelques fonctions involontaires des appareils de la locomotion de la prehension et de la voix. Archives of General Medicine 1825; 8:385–407; and Guilly P. Gilles de la Tourette. In Rose FC, Bynum WF (eds), *Historical Aspects of the Neurosciences*. New York: Raven Press, 1982, pp397–413.

5   A drug that blocks the action of the neurotransmitter dopamine in the brain, and known to be effective in controlling the symptoms of Tourette's. Haloperidol is more commonly used as an antipsychotic drug.

6   Freud is not known to have written on tic disorders or coprolalia.

7   Otto Fenichel (1897–1946) was a member of the Viennese Psychoanalytical Association as a young man and attended Freud's lectures during his medical school training. He was also influenced by Marxist theory and proposed that psychoanalysis would be at the core of a future dialectical materialism. Fenichel O. *The Psychoanalytic Theory of Neurosis*. New York: Norton & Co. 1945.

8   Popper K. *Conjectures and Refutations: The Growth of Scientific Knowledge*. New York: Harper & Row, 1968, pp34–5. Sir Karl Popper (1902–94) is regarded as one of the most influential philosophers of science of the twentieth century. He was also a social and political philosopher and a staunch defender of the open society.

9   A study of a worldwide sample of 488 societies revealed that altered states of consciousness occurred in almost all societies, and 52 per cent associated these alterations with spirit possession.

10 Shapiro AK, Shapiro ES, Young JG, Feinberg TE. *Gilles de la Tourette Syndrome*. New York: Raven Press 1988.

11 Andrey Andreyevich Markov (1856–1922) was a Russian mathematician who developed the theory of stochastic processes, especially those called Markov chains.

12 Nuwer MR. Coprolalia as an organic symptom. Advances in Neurology 1982; 35: 363–8.

13 Wohlfart G, Ingvar DH, Hellberg AM. Compulsory shouting (Benedek's

'klazomania') associated with oculogyric spasms in chronic epidemic encephalitis. Acta Psychiatrica Scandinavica 1961; 36:369–77.

14 Shapiro AK, Shapiro ES. Tic disorders. In Kaplan HI, Sadock BJ (eds), *Comprehensive Textbook of Psychiatry V*. Baltimore: Williams & Wilkins 1989, pp1865–78 (quote from p1869).

15 Sacks OW. Neuropsychiatry and Tourette's. In Mueller J (ed.), *Neurology and Psychiatry: A Meeting of Minds*. Basel: Karger 1989, p164.

4   The Mozart complex

1   Farah MJ, Illes J, Cook-Deegan R et al. Neurocognitive enhancement: What can we do and what should we do? Nature Reviews Neuroscience 2004; 5:421–5.

2   Canton J. Designing the future: NBIC technologies and human performance enhancement. Ann NY Acad Sci 2004; 1013:186–98.

3   Giurgea C. Vers une pharmacologie de l activité integrative du cerveau. Tentative du concept nootrope en psychpharmacolgie (Pharmacology of integrative activity of the brain. Attempt at nootropic concept in psychopharmacology). Actual Pharmacol (Paris) 1972, 25: 115–56.

4   Schaffler K, Klausnitzer W. Antihypoxidotic effects of Piracetam using psychophysiological measures in healthy volunteers. Ar Forsch. Drug Res. 1988; 38:288–91.

5   Clement BA, Goff E, Burt CM, Forbes T, David A. Toxic amines and alkaloids from Acacia berlandieri. Phytochemistry 1997; 46(2):249–54. A year later another Acacia species (*A. rigidula*) was found to have amphetamine.

6   Borowsky B et al. Trace amines: Identification of a family of mammalian G protein-coupled receptors. Proc Natl Acad Sci USA 2001; 98:8966–71.

7   Elliott R, Sahakian BJ, Matthews K et al. Effects of methylphenidate on spatial working memory and planning in healthy young adults. Psychopharmacology 1997; 131:196–206.

8   Mehta MA, Owen AM, Sahakian BJ et al. Methylphenidate enhances working memory by modulating discrete frontal and parietal lobe regions in the human brain. J Neurosci 2000; 20:RC65.

9   Turner DC, Robbins TW, Luke C, Aron AR, Dowson J, Sahakian BJ. Cognitive enhancing effects of modafinil in healthy volunteers. Psychopharmacology 165 (3):260–9.

10 Caldwell JA, Caldwell JL, Smith JK, Brown DL, 'Modafinil's effects on simulator performance and mood in pilots during 37 hours without sleep. Aviation, Space, and Environmental Medicine 2004, 75:777–84. Caldwell JA, Caldwell JL. Fatigue in military aviation: An overview of US

military-approved pharmacological countermeasures. Aviation, Space, and Environmental Medicine, 2005, 76 (7):39–51.

11   Wong D, Horng J, Bymaster F, Hauser K, Molloy B. A selective inhibitor of serotonin uptake: Lilly 110140, 3-(p-trifluoromethylphenoxy)-N-methyl-3-phenylpropylamine. Life Sci 1974; 15(3):471–9.

12   Carlsson A, Wong DT. A note on the discovery of selective serotonin reuptake inhibitors. Life Sci 1997; 61(12):1203.

13   Kramer PD. *Listening to Prozac*. New York: Penguin, 1993.

14   Dean W, Morgenthaler J. *Smart Drugs and Nutrients*. Santa Cruz, CA: B & J Publications, 1991.

15   Solomon PR, Adams F, Silver A, et al. Ginkgo for memory enhancement: A randomized controlled trial. Journal of the American Medical Association 2002; 288(7):835–40.

16   Yesavage J, Mumenthaler M, Taylor J, et al. Donepezil and flight simulator performance: Effects on retention of complex skills. Neurology 2001; 59:123–5.

17   Lynch G. Memory enhancement: The search for mechanism-based drugs. Nat Neurosci Suppl 2003; 5:1035–8.

18   Miller, BL, Ponton, M, Benson, DF, Cummings, JL, Mena, I. Enhanced artistic creativity with temporal lobe degeneration. Lancet. 1996; 348(9043):1744–5.

19   Mell JC, Howard SM, Miller BL. Art and the brain: The influence of fronto-temporal dementia on an accomplished artist. Neurology 2003; 60:1707–10.

20   Rankin KP, Liu AA, Howard S, Slama H, Hou CE, Shuster K, Miller BL. A case-controlled study of altered visual art production in Alzheimer's and FTLD. Cognitive & Behavioral Neurology 2007, 20(1):48–61.

21   Snyder AW, Mulcahy E, Taylor JL, Mitchell DJ, Sachdev P, Gandevia SC. Savant-like skills exposed in normal people by suppressing the left fronto-temporal lobe. Journal of Integrative Neuroscience 2003; 2:149–58.

5   The mirror always lies

1   Coming face to face with this statue at the Accademia in Florence, after a two-hour wait in the heat, was one of my most joyous and awe-inspiring moments. Only the first sight of the Taj Mahal evoked a similar emotion.

2   Ironically, anorexia is often referred to by the shorthand 'ana' on the internet.

3   Lanugo are fine hairs that are present on the foetus but are lost at 36–40 weeks of gestation. When present on a newborn, they indicate prematurity.

Lanugo hairs appear in anorexia and are considered to be the body's response to loss of fat as an attempt at insulation.

4   BMI (body mass index) is a measure of body fat based on height and weight. The normal range is 20 to 25. BMI of 15 or less usually warrants hospitalisation; 10–12 is the lower limit of survival.

5   This belief of the individual has been called an 'overvalued idea' rather than a delusion. While it is a fixed, false belief, invested with considerable emotion, it may unfortunately be shared in some cases, or is an extreme version of what may be considered normal. The boundary between overvalued ideas and delusions is sometimes blurred. For example, when sexual jealousy or religious fervour becomes a delusion is often debated by psychiatrists.

6   These techniques were reviewed in an excellent paper by S Skrzypek and colleagues from Germany (Body image assessment using body size estimation in recent studies on anorexia nervosa. A brief review. Eur Child Adolesc Psychiatry 2001; 10(4):215–21).

7   Her book *The Golden Cage: The Enigma of Anorexia Nervosa* (Cambridge, MA: Harvard University Press, 1978) is possibly the best lay introduction to this fascinating disorder.

8   This increase in blood supply to a brain region that needs it more is an automatic process, much like the increase of blood supply to an active muscle.

9   Ellison Z et al. Functional anatomy of calorie fear in anorexia nervosa. Lancet 1998; 352:1192.

10 Durston S et al. Anatomical MRI of the developing human brain: What have we learned? J Am Acad Child Adolesc Psychiatry 2001; 40:1012–20.

11 The neurologist Antonio Damasio has proposed that it is the area of brain representation of the states of bodily organs in relation to emotion – it is the cognitive representation of the body and gives rise to conscious feeling about the body. The insula is also involved in food and drug craving.

12 Anna Freud (1895–1982) was the youngest child of Sigmund Freud and the only one to follow her father's footsteps in developing psychoanalytic theory. She is known for her work on the ego and her concepts of development in early childhood. Her most widely read work is *The Ego and the Mechanisms of Defence* (New York: International Universities Press, 1966).

13 Stroke in the right cerebral hemisphere leads to weakness on the left side due to crossing over of the motor fibres as they travel through the brain stem down to the spinal cord.

14 Babinski was one of the many distinguished pupils of the great French

neurologist Charcot, who worked at the Salpêtrière in Paris in late nineteenth century. (Hôpital de la Salpêtrière has an important place in the history of neurology. Charcot's legendary clinical demonstrations took place in the exalted halls of this institution.) Babinski was a keen clinical observer and achieved eponymous fame for his discovery of the plantar reflex (Babinski's sign) and a number of neurological syndromes.

15 Marcel A, Tegner R, Nimmo-Smith I. Anosognosia for plegia: Specificity, extension, partiality and disunity of bodily unawareness. Cortex 2004; 40:19–40.

16 The Wada test is named after Juhn A. Wada, a Canadian neuropsychologist, who worked with Wilder Penfield and Brenda Milner at Montreal Neurological Institute. It was ostensibly to help Penfield better lateralise language function in the brain before surgery.

17 Gilmore RL, Heilman KM, Schmidt RP, Fennell EM, Quisling R. Anosognosia during Wada test. Neurology 1992; 42:925–7.

18 Ramachandran VS, Rogers-Ramachandran D. Denial of disabilities in anosognosia. Nature 1996; 382:501.

19 Gusnard DA et al. Medial prefrontal cortex and self-referential mental activity: Relation to a default mode of brain function. PNAS 2001; 98:4259–64.

20 Premack DG, Woodruff G. Does the chimpanzee have a theory of mind? Behavioral and Brain Sciences, 1978; 1:515–26.

6 The dead homunculus

1 Tilney F. *The Brain, from Ape to Man*. New York: Hoeber, 1928.

2 Homunculi, the little people in the brain, are explored by Daniel Dennett in his book *Brainstorms* (Montgomery, VT: Bradford Books, 1978). This book contains some of the most lucid discussions on issues confronting philosophers of the mind.

3 Herman Boerhaave is often regarded as the founder of clinical teaching and the modern academic hospital. He made the University of Leiden famous for its clinical teaching, and is said to have taught Peter the Great and been visited by Linnaeus and Voltaire.

4 Kaplan GA [1899]. Cited in: Van Hasselt VB, Hersen M (eds). *Handbook of Psychological Approaches with Violent Offenders: Contemporary Strategies and Issues*. Birhäuser, 1999.

5 Monroe RR. Maturational lag in central nervous system development as a partial explanation of episodic violent behavior. Psychopharmacol Bull. 1974, 10(4):63–4.

6 Mark V, Ervin F. *Violence and the Brain*, Hagerstown, MD: Harper & Row,

1970. The book proved very controversial because of the extension of the organic theories of violent behaviour to social violence. Drawing attention to the fact that in riots only a few individuals got hurt, they suggested that 'it would be particularly interesting under these circumstances to examine in detail those individuals who did cause serious injury or death – be they rioters or members of the police and National Guard' (pp151–2). Even more controversial was the recommendation of 'newer techniques in the diagnosis and treatment of violent patients' (p159), including brain surgery.

7   Brickner RM. *The Intellectual Functions of the Frontal Lobes*. New York: Macmillan, 1936.

8   Egas Moniz (1874–1953) was a Portuguese neurologist who is best known for introducing neurosurgery for the treatment of psychiatric disorders, also called psychosurgery, for which he was awarded the Nobel Prize for Medicine in 1949.

9   The 'happiness cult' refers to the Church of God movement started in the 1920s by Elder Solomon Lightfoot Michaux in Philadelphia, which had the theme song 'Happy Am I'.

10 The first famous patient with frontal lobe damage, who provides an excellent description of the associated complex behavioural disturbance, was Phineas Gage (also known as the Boston Crowbar Case), described by Harlow in the 1880s. Harlow HF, Harlow MK, Suomi SJ. From thought to therapy: Lessons from a primate laboratory. American Scientist. 1971, 59(5):538–49.

11 The National Adult Reading Test (NART), or a person's reading ability, is not generally affected by brain injury, and reflects intellectual and educational abilities, allowing it to be used to assess the level before the injury.

12 Alexander Luria (1902–77) was a Russian neuropsychologist who is best recognised in neurology for his method of observation of neuropsychological patients. His two detailed descriptions of patients are famous: *Mind of a Mnemonist* and *The Man with a Shattered World*. He is regarded as one of the founders of cultural–historical psychology.

13 MRI uses powerful magnets and the magnetic properties of charged particles such as protons in the brain, to construct pictures of the living brain in exquisite anatomical detail. It has produced a veritable revolution in the study of the structural basis of neurological disease.

14 Sir Karl Popper and Sir John Eccles, *The Self and Its Brain*. Sir Karl Popper (1902–94) was one of the most influential philosophers of science of the twentieth century. His book *The Logic of Scientific Discovery* (London: Routledge, 1959; new edition 2002) was a landmark event.

He co-authored *The Self and Its Brain* with Sir John Eccles in 1977 as an argument for interactionism (Routledge, reprint edition, 1984).

15 Robert Nozick (1938–2002) was an analytical philosopher at Harvard University who published influential works on knowledge, free will, personal identity, the nature of value and the meaning of life.

16 The model of the frontal lobes as the supervisory system is best expounded by Tim Shallice in his book *From Neuropsychology to Mental Structure* (Cambridge: Cambridge University Press, 1988), which is greatly influenced by Fodor's modularity thesis of brain function.

17 Hofstadter DR. Can creativity be mechanized? Scientific American 1982; 247:18–34. Hofstadter calls the insect-like stereotyped behaviour 'sphexishness'.

18 An excellent description of this is provided in a recent review: Iacoboni M, Dapretto M. The mirror neuron system and the consequences of its dysfunction. Nature Reviews Neuroscience 2006; 7:942–51.

19 For an excellent account of this, please see Arbib M. From monkey-like action recognition to human language: An evolutionary framework for neurolinguistics. Behavioral and Brain Sciences 2005; 28:105–67.

20 Empathy is the ability to perceive and feel directly the emotion of another person. It is not to be confused with sympathy or compassion.

21 Wicker B, Keysers C, Plailly J, Royet JP, Gallese V, Rizzolatti G. Both of us disgusted in my insula: The common neural basis of seeing and feeling disgust. Neuron. 2003; 40(3):655–64.

22 Iacoboni M et al. Grasping the intentions of others with one's own mirror neuron system. PLoS Biol 2005; 3:e79. This was an fMRI study that showed that the response was different in the mirror neuron system depending upon the context in which the action was embedded.

7 Serotonin's seductive song

1 Charles Darwin (1809–82) is widely regarded as the most important naturalist of modern times. His theory of evolution formed the basis of modern biology. His 1859 book *On the Origin of Species* revolutionised our thinking by establishing evolution by common descent as the dominant scientific explanation for the occurrence of the large number of species in nature and the basis of human evolution. He developed his theories further in *The Descent of Man and in Selection in Relation to Sex*, followed by *The Expression of the Emotions in Man and Animals* in 1872. The last book contains many sketches and photographs of animals and humans expressing various emotions.

2 William James (1842–1910) is regarded as one of the most significant

psychologists of the late nineteenth and twentieth centuries. His monumental work *The Principles of Psychology* (1890) has influenced generations of psychologists and philosophers. His essay 'What is an emotion?' appeared in *Mind* in 1884. He was a brilliant writer as well, and it has been quipped that William was the better writer and his brother Henry (famous for such works as *Portrait of a Lady*) the better psychologist.

3   Lange C in Dunlap E (ed.). *The Emotions.* Baltimore, MD: Williams & Wilkins, 1885, pp33–90.

4   Cannon, WB. The James–Lange theory of emotions: A critical examination and an alternative theory. Am J Psychol 1927; 39:106–24. Cannon, WB. Against the James–Lange and the thalamic theories of emotions. Psychol Rev 1931; 38:281–95.

5   Acknowledging the contribution of the psychologist Philip Bard.

6   The hypothalamus, literally below the thalamus, is an almond-sized brain region that controls body temperature, hunger, thirst and circadian rhythms. It is linked to the limbic system, which controls emotions and sexual behaviour.

7   Ekman P, Levenson RW, Friesen, W Autonomic nervous system activity distinguishes among emotions. Science 1983; 221:1208–10.

8   Hess W. In *Physiology or Medicine 1942–1962*, Nobel Lectures, Amsterdam: Elsevier, 1964.

9   'Affect' is the technical term for the outwardly displayed mood. The use of this term recognises the fact that the outward display of emotion might not necessarily reveal what the individual is feeling inside. Since one will never know what a cat is feeling inside, it is accurate to refer to the display as 'affective'.

10   Depression is one of the disorders of affect. Sano M, Yoshioka M, Ogashiwa B, Ishijima C, Ohye C. Postero-medial hypothalamotomy in the treatment of aggressive behaviors. Stereotactic and Functional Neurosurgery 1966; 27:164–7 (DOI: 10.1159/000103949). From the Department of Neurosurgery, Faculty of Medicine, University of Tokyo.

11   Papez JW. A proposed mechanism of emotion. 1937. Reprinted in J Neuropsychiatry Clin Neurosci. 1995; 7(1):103–12.

12   Bush G, Luu P, Posner MI. Cognitive and emotional influences in anterior cingulate cortex. Trends Cognit Sci 2000; 4:215–22.

13   The region stimulated was Brodmann area 25 (Cg25).

14   Mayberg HS, Lozano AM, Voon V, McNeely HE, Seminowicz D, Hamani C et al. Deep brain stimulation for treatment-resistant depression. Neuron 2005; 45(5):651–60 (quote from p652).

15   Weiskrantz L. Behavioral changes associated with ablation of the

amygdaloid complex in monkeys. J Comp Physiol Psychol 1956; 49:381–91.

16 Paul Pierre Broca (1824–80) was a notable French physician, anatomist and anthropologist who is best remembered in medicine for his discovery of the speech production area in the brain (known as Broca's area), which started a series of studies into localisation of brain function.

17 An excellent exposition of the neuroanatomy of emotional behaviour can be found by the book by Dr J LeDoux, *The Emotional Brain*, New York: Simon & Schuster, 1996. Another account is in the article LeDoux JE. Emotion, memory and the brain. Sci Am 1994; 270:50–7. An article that might appeal to the neuroscientist is LeDoux JE. Emotion circuits in the brain. Annu Rev Neurosci 2000; 23:155–84.

18 A good review of their and related work: Rauch SL, Shin LM, Phelps EA. Neurocircuitry models of posttraumatic stress disorder and extinction: Human neuroimaging research – past, present, and future. Biol Psychiatry 2006; 60(4):376–82.

19 Bechara A, Tranel D, Damasio H, Adolphs R, Rockland C, Damasio AR. Double dissociation of conditioning and declarative knowledge relative to the amygdala and hippocampus in humans. Science 1995; 269(5227):1115–18.

20 Appropriately referred to as the insular cortex – it is also called the Island of Reil, after Johann Christian Reil.

21 The insula is central to Antonio Damasio's somatic marker hypothesis.

22 Lazar SW, Kerr CE, Wasserman RH, Gray JR, Greve DN, Treadway MT et al. Meditation experience is associated with increased cortical thickness. NeuroReport 2005; 16(17):1893–7.

23 Damasio referred at Elliott as the modern Phineas Gage. The story of Gage is an interesting one. One of the landmark cases in neuropsychology, he suffered a horrific injury to his frontal lobes when an iron rod traversed the front of his head. His case was studied in detail by Dr JM Harlow and provided some of the early insights into the functions of the frontal lobes. Harlow JM. Passage of an iron rod through the head. Boston Medical and Surgical Journal 1848–49; 39:389.

24 The Mayer–Salovey model has been highly influential. Mayer JD, Salovey P. The intelligence of emotional intelligence. Intelligence 1993; 17:433–42.

25 Goleman D. *Emotional Intelligence: Why It Can Matter More Than IQ*. London: Bloomsbury, 1996.

26 Premack DG, Woodruff G. Does the chimpanzee have a theory of mind? Behavioral and Brain Sciences 1978; 1:515–26.

27 Price JS, Sloman L, Gardner R, Gilbert P, Rhode P. The social competition

hypothesis of depression. British Journal of Psychiatry 1994; 164:309–15.

28 Keller MC, Nesse, RM. Is low mood an adaptation? Evidence for subtypes with symptoms that match precipitants. Journal of Affective Disorders 2005; 86:27–35.

29 This topic has been reviewed by a number of authors. For some recent reviews, see: Sheline YI. Neuroimaging studies of mood disorder effect on the brain. Biol Psychiatry 2003; 54:338–52, and Rogers MA et al. Executive and prefrontal dysfunction in unipolar depression: A review of neuropsychological ad imaging evidence. Neurosci Res 2004; 50:1–11.

30 They were previously called the corpus striatum – originally identified by the great anatomist Thomas Willis in 1664.

31 Alexander GE, DeLong MR, Strick PL. Parallel organisation of functionally segregated circuits linking basal ganglia and cortex. Annual Review of Neuroscience 1986; 9:357–81.

32 This is unlike schizophrenic patients, who are unable to activate their prefrontal cortex to the normal level.

33 For further description of this chemical, refer to chapter 8 of this book.

34 There are different theories as to how a large carbohydrate meal might cause drowsiness. An older explanation relates to blood being diverted to the stomach and away from the brain. The more likely explanation is that carbohydrate induces release of insulin, which diverts large neutral-branched amino acids, but not tryptophan, into protein synthesis and increases the relative levels of tryptophan in the blood and thereby the brain. It is therefore the potatoes, squash, pumpkin pie and bread from the meal that cause the 'turkey coma', but tryptophan does end up playing some part.

35 For a recent review of this field, see Ruhé HG, Mason NS, Schene AH. Mood is indirectly related to serotonin, norepinephrine and dopamine levels in humans: A meta-analysis of monoamine depletion studies. Molecular Psychiatry 2007; 12:331–59.

36 Marketed by Servier in France.

37 It bears worth repeating that nerve cells are not continuous with one another – there is a gap between the axon of one cell and the body of another cell, which is called the synapse. The chemical messenger traverses this synapse to convey information between the two cells.

38 See Mitchell AJ. Two-week delay in the onset of action of antidepressants: New evidence. British Journal of Psychiatry 2006; 188:105–6.

39 Arvid Carlsson (b. 1923) is a Swedish neuroscientist who was awarded the Nobel Prize in Physiology and Medicine (with Eric Kandel and Paul Greengard) in 2000 for his work on dopamine as a neurotransmitter. His

discovery led to the treatment of Parkinson's disease with L–dopa.

40 Carlsson A. A half-century of neurotransmitter research: Impact on neurology and psychiatry. Nobel Lecture 8 Dec 2000. <http://nobelprize.org/nobel_prizes/medicine/laurates/2000/carlsson-lecture.pdf>

41 Nibuya M, Morinobu S, Duman RS. Regulation of BDNF and trkB mRNA in rat brain by chronic electroconvulsive seizure and antidepressant drug treatments. Journal of Neuroscience 1995; 15:7539–47.

42 One measure of the genetic contribution is 'heritability', which is a statement on the amount of variation of a particular phenomenon is accounted for by genetic factors. Twin and family genetic studies are conducted to determine this. A review of the evidence for major depressive disorder was published recently: Sullivan PF, Neale MC, Kendler KS. Genetic epidemiology of major depression: Review and meta-analysis. Am J Psychiatry 2000; 157(10):1552–62.

43 Caspi A, Sugden K, Moffitt TE et al. Influence of life stress on depression: Moderation by a polymorphism in the 5-HTT gene. Science 2003; 301(5631):386–9.

8 A chesty problem

1 Rapoport J. *The Boy Who Couldn't Stop Washing*. London: Fontana, 1989.

2 Morris D, *The Naked Ape*. NY: McGraw-Hill, 1967. Desmond Morris is a well-known zoologist and ethnologist, a popular writer and television presenter, as well as an artist in the surrealist tradition. He explained human behaviour from his zoological perspective, through an evolutionary lens. Many of his theories have been criticised as being incomplete or unscientific. *The Naked Ape* is his best-known book, but he has been a prolific people-watcher and writer.

3 Cant J. Hypothesis for the evolution of human breasts and buttocks. American Naturalist 1981; 117:199–204.

4 Mascia-Lees FE, Relethford J, Sorger T. Evolutionary perspectives on permanent breast enlargement in human females. American Anthropologist 1986; 88:423–8.

5 The MRI scanner creates an image of the the brain using the electromagnetic properties of H+ nuclei or protons, so abundant in brain tissue and cerebrospinal fluid. Some MRI scan differences between OCD patients and healthy comparison individuals have been described, but these relate to group comparisons and cannot be translated to the individual patient.

6 PET for positron emission tomography. The most commonly used PET scan examines the rate of glucose uptake by different brain regions,

using 18F-deoxyglucose (FDG). Since glucose is the exclusive fuel for neurons, this gives the metabolic rate of different brain regions. Rates of metabolism might be abnormal in regions that are structurally normal.

7   Sachdev P, Trollor J, Walker A, Wen W, Fulham M, Smith JS et al. Bilateral orbitomedial leucotomy for obsessive compulsive disorder: A single case study using positron emission tomography. Aust NZ J Psychiatry 2001; 35(5):684–90.

8   Pierre Marie Félix Janet, French physician, psychiatrist and philosopher, born 30 May 1859, Paris; died 24 February 1947, Paris. He was influential in bringing academic psychology and treatment of mental disorders together. He is best known for his work on hysteria. He worked with Jean-Martin Charcot, just like Sigmund Freud.

9   Janet believed that psychological tension related to 'some physiological tension' in the central nervous system. Displacement was a kind of diversion of mental energy.

10 Freud divided the stages of development of childhood sexuality into oral, anal and genetic stages. Fixation at or regression to a particular stage later in life led to certain personality characteristics or neuroses.

11 Rapport MM, Green AA, Page IH. Serum vasoconstrictor (serotonin). IV. Isolation and characterization. J Biol Chem 1948; 176(3):1243–51.

9   Lord Nelson's ghost

1   Jeffery W (ed.). *The Naval Chronicle 1798–1818*, 40 vols. <http://nla.gov. au/nla.aus-vn2255604>

2   This is quoted from Riddoch G. Phantom limbs and body shape. Brain 1941; 64:197–222.

3   Mitchell first described this phenomenon in soldiers during the Civil War in the USA (Mitchell SW. Phantom limbs. Lippincott's Magazine for Popular Literature and Science 1871; 8:563–9). Not unlike Julian, Dr Mitchell was anxious about the reactions in the scientific community to his descriptions of phantom limbs, and chose to publish his findings in a popular lay journal. His observations were astute and have been confirmed by hundreds of investigators. Dr Silas Weir Mitchell (1829–1914) is a colourful figure in the history of neurology, and is best remembered for his descriptions of 'causalgia', erythromelalgia and post-paralytic chorea, which established a firm place for him in medicine.

4   See Zuk's paper for a psychodynamic interpretation. Zuk GH. The phantom limb: A proposed theory of unconscious origins. J Nerv Ment Dis 1956; 124:510–13.

5   Melzack is one of the foremost experts on pain. His views on the phantom

limb are summarised in the paper Melzack R. Phantom limbs and the concept of a neuromatrix. Trends in Neuroscience 1990; 13:88–92.

6   Dr Ramachandran has written an intriguing book, *Phantoms in the Brain* (Ramachandran VS, Blakeslee S. London: Fourth Estate, 1998), which presents a detailed account of phantom limbs (and breasts, penises, etc) along with his remarkable experiments conducted with a creative simplicity not commonly seen in scientific investigators these days. His brilliant work guided my own approach to this patient.

7   Ramachandran VS, Hirstein W. The perception of phantom limbs: The DO Hebb lecture. Brain 1998; 121:1603–30.

8   For a more detailed exposition of this, see ibid.

9   Much of the earlier information about this comes from the work of the Canadian neurosurgeon Dr Wilder Penfield, who mapped this in his patients on the surgical table. See Penfield W, Rasmussen TL. *The Cerebral Cortex of Man: A Clinical Study of Localization of Function*. New York: Macmillan, 1950.

10   Merzenich MM, Nelson RJ, Stryker MP et al. Somatosensory cortical map changes following digit amputation in adult monkeys. J Comp Neurol 1984; 224:591–605.

11   Pons TP, Garraghty PE, Ommaya AK et al. Massive cortical reorganization after sensory deafferentation in adult macaques. Science 1991; 252:1857–60.

12   Yang T, Gallen C, Ramachandran VS, Schwartz BJ, Bloom FE. Noninvasive detection of cerebral plasticity in adult human somatosensory cortex. Neuroreport 1994; 5:701–4.

13   Weinstein S, Sersen EA, Vetter RJ. Phantoms and somatic sensations in cases of congenital aplasia. Cortex 1964; 1:276–90.

14   See Gentili ME, Verton C, Kinirons B, Bonnet F. Clinical perception of phantom limb sensation in patients with brachial plexus block. Eur J Anaesthesiol. 2002; 19(2):105–8.

15   Sunderland S. *Nerves and Nerve Injuries*. 2nd edn. Edinburgh: Churchill Livingstone, 1978.

16   The medical term is pseudocyesis (literally, false pregnancy).

17   Ramachandran VS. Behavioral and magnetoencephalographic correlates of plasticity in the adult human brain. Proceedings of the National Academy of Science USA 1993; 90:10413–20.

18   Ramachandran VS, Rogers-Ramachandran D. Synaesthesia in phantom limbs induced with mirrors. Proceedings of the Royal Society, London, part B. 1996; 263:377–86.

19   Ramachandran VS, Rogers-Ramachandran D, Cobb S. Touching the

phantom limb. Nature. 1995; 377(6549):489–90.

20 Ancient Indian philiosophy refers to this as *maya* (literally 'not that'), according to which the 'reality' of the universe is a fleeting illusion , which must be seen through for enlightenment to be attained.

10 Freudian slips and semantic slides

1 An excellent account of the tip-of-the-tongue (TOT) phenomenon can be found in Schwartz BL. Tip-of-the-tongue phenomenon: Gold mine or can of worms? Mahwah, NJ: Lawrence Erlbaum, 2002. A caveat! Schwartz draws a great deal from laboratory-induced TOTs, which differ from the TOTs of everyday life. An interesting reference in these experiments is to 'illusory' TOTs, i.e. TOTs for unanswerable questions (e.g. what is the capital of Bormea?)

2 William James, in his 1890 classic *The Principles of Psychology* (New York: Dover, 1950), gave an excellent description of the 'gap' in knowing. 'Suppose we try to recall a forgotten name ... there is a gap therein; but no mere gap. It is a gap that is intensely active. A sort of a wraith of a name is in it, beckoning us in a given direction ... If the wrong names are proposed to us this singular gap acts immediately so as to negate them ... And the gap of one word does not feel like the gap of another, all empty of content as both might seem necessarily to be when described as gaps ... There are innumerable consciousness of emptiness, no one of which taken in itself has a name, but all different from each other' (pp251–2).

3 Burke DM et al. On the tip of the tongue: What causes word-finding failures in young and older adults. Journal of Memory and Language 1991; 30:542–79.

4 Thompson R, Emmorey K, Gollan TH. 'Tip of the fingers' experiences of deaf signers. Psychological Science 2005; 16:856–60.

5 Damasio A. *Descartes' Error: Emotion, Reason, and the Human Brain*, New York: Putnam Publishing, 1994.

6 Freud S. *Psychopathology of Everyday Life*. 1901. AA Brill (trans.) 1914. From the Classics in the History of Psychology. <http://psychclassics.yorku.ca/Freud/Psycho> An internet resource developed by Christopher D Green, York University, Toronto, Ontario.

7 'Semantics' refers to meaning in language whereas 'phonological' refers to sounds.

8. Diamond J, *The Third Chimpanzee: The Evolution and Future of the Human Animal*. New York: Harper Perennial, 1992, 2006, pp141–67.

9 Kanzi was a Bonobo (Pygmy Chimpanzee, *Pan paniscus*) who was studied

by Sue Savage-Rumbaugh, a primatologist from Georgia State University, Atlanta, GA. It is believed that Kanzi understood more human language than any other nonhuman animal in the world. An interesting story often related is that the researcher one day wrote a sentence on the computer that Kanzi had never heard before: 'Can you make the dog bite the snake?' Kanzi is said to have selected a toy dog and a toy snake from the objects available and put the snake in the dog's mouth. When 7½ years old, Kanzi is said to have had an accuracy of 74 per cent in responding to 600 complex questions. The language ability of apes of which Savage-Rumbaugh was a strong proponent was strongly criticised by many linguists and neuroscientists, including Steven Pinker. Savage-Rumbaugh ES, McDonald K, Sevcik RA, Hopkins WD, Rupert E. Spontaneous symbol acquisition and communicative use by pygmy chimpanzees (*Pan paniscus*). Journal of Experimental Psychology: General 1986; 115:211–35.

10 Proto-language has a 'me Tarzan, you Jane' quality about it.

11 The neocortex is the newest part of the cerebral cortex, the outer layer of the brain that is involved in higher mental functions. Compared to other primates, the neocortex has vastly expanded in humans.

12 Papagno C, Capitani E. Proper name anomia: A case with sparing of the first-letter knowledge. Neuropsychologia. 1998; 36(7):669–79.

13 Ibid.

14 Fronto-temporal dementias (FTD) are a group of disorders with progressive atrophy of the frontal and/or temporal lobes, with eventual involvement of the entire cortex. Patients with FTD often present with behavioural symptoms or language difficulties rather than pure memory problems. Pick's disease is one type of FTD. Patients with right temporal lobe lesions may also develop the phenomenon of prosopagnosia, or an inability to recognise or put names to faces.

15 Evans JJ, Heggs AJ, Antoun N, Hodges JR. Progressive prosopagnosia associated with selective right temporal lobe atrophy: A new syndrome? Brain 1995; 118:1–13.

16 McKenna P, Warrington EK. Category-specific naming preservation: a single case study. J Neurol Neurosurg Psychiatry 1978; 41:571–4.

17 Nielsen JM. *Agnosia, Apraxia, Aphasia: Their Value in Cerebral Localization*, 2nd edn. New York: Hoeber, 1946.

18 Warrington EK, Shallice T. Category specific semantic impairments. Brain 1984; 107:829–53.

19 Crutch SJ, Ridha BH, Warrington EK. The different frameworks underlying abstract and concrete knowledge: Evidence from a bilingual patient with a semantic refractory access dysphasia. Neurocase 2006;

12:151–63.

20 Paradis M. *Assessment of Bilingual Aphasia*. Hillsdale, NJ: Lawrence Erlbaum, 1987.

21 Mendez MF, Perryman KM, Ponton MO, Cummings JL. Bilingualism and dementia. J Neuropsychiatry Clin Neuroscience 1999; 11:411–12.

22 This work was carried out by researchers at Rotman Research Institute, Toronto, Canada. They examined 184 patients who attended Ross Memory Clinic between 2002 and 2005, of whom 91 were monolingual and 93 were bilingual, the latter including speakers of 25 different languages, predominantly Eastern European. The mean age of onset of dementia in the monolinguals was 71.4 years and in the bilinguals 75.5 years.

23 Page TL, Einstein M, Duan H et al. Morphological alterations in neurons forming corticortical projections in the neocortex of aged patas monkeys. Neurosci Lett 2001; 317:37–41.

Index